ATHEROMA

Atherosclerosis in
Ischaemic Heart Disease:
The Mechanisms

ATHEROMA

Atherosclerosis in Ischaemic Heart Disease:

Volume 1 The Mechanisms

M J Davies MD MRCP FRCPath

Professor of Cardiovascular Pathology
St George's Hospital Medical School, London

N Woolf PhD MMed (Path) FRCPath

Bland Sutton Professor of Histopathology
University College and Middlesex School of Medicine
University College, London

Presented as a service to cardiology
by Bayer UK Limited

Bayer C·A·R·E

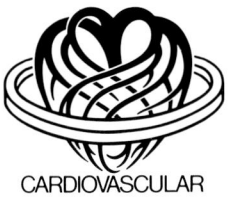

CARDIOVASCULAR

Copyright © 1990 by Science Press Limited
6 Lowther Road
London SW13 9ND

British Library Cataloguing in Publication Data
   Atheroma
   Vol 1
   1. Man. Cardiovascular system. Diseases
   I. Davies, M.J. (Michael John) II. Woolf, Neville
   616.1
ISBN 1-870026-31-4
ISBN 1-870026-41-1 set
ISBN 1-870026-36-5 V.2

Edited by Sharyn Wong
Designed by Robin Dodd FCSD
Linework by Lynda Payne
Printed in Spain by Imago Publishing Limited

FOREWORD

Atherosclerosis remains the predominant disease of most developed countries and is the most common cause of disability and death amongst wealthier populations, mainly through involvement of the coronary and carotid arteries. The validity of this generalization has not been impaired by the decreasing incidence of coronary heart disease in the United States, where it has dropped by approximately 30% since the 1960s. The reason for this exceptional downward trend remains obscure, but it is a hopeful indication that there is a possibility of arresting and reversing the increases in coronary heart disease that are still occurring in several other countries.

The reason for high prevalences of atherosclerotic diseases is, however, now known. Epidemiological evidence has established a direct relationship between coronary heart disease and cholesterol levels in the diet and in plasma. There is no longer any doubt that atherosclerosis begins with focal accumulations of plasma lipids, mainly cholesterol, in the form of plasma low-density lipoprotein (LDL) in the intima of arteries, which differ in their susceptibility to this process. Elucidation of the atherogenic effect of LDL and of its control by a specific cellular receptor, for which the Nobel Prize was awarded to J. L. Goldstein and M. S. Brown, was a major advance in understanding the mechanisms at work in the disease.

This volume is concerned with the mechanisms of atheroma, and another mechanism about which knowledge is rapidly increasing, that which frequently marks the end of the disease, myocardial infarction. There was the question of the immediate cause of this striking clinical event, which is almost always sudden and unpredictable. The answer was provided by M. J. Davies, who has contributed a chapter to this volume, whose quantitative reconstructions of atherosclerotic coronary arteries established the connexion of myocardial infarction with plaque fissuring leading to intramural haemorrhage and thrombus formation.

This major step forward, since confirmed by E. Falk and others, has led to a systemic analysis of the properties of human plaques which may make them liable to fissuring. Recently, P. D. Richardson, M. J. Davies and I have provided evidence by computer modelling that regions of high circumferential stress correlate well with the sites of intimal fissures found *post mortem*. Furthermore, histological observations show that the sites of fissures are influenced by variations in the mechanical strength of plaque caps related to focal accumulation of foam cells. This suggests that local weak points in caps may account for fissures away from points of maximum stress.

It is appropriate that the mechanisms responsible for atherosclerosis should be here considered by M. J. Davies and N. Woolf, two distinguished pathologists who have exceptional experience in this disease. In order to avoid 'red herrings' in the future, which have been plentiful in the past, it is essential that research into pathogenesis should never lose sight of the actual human lesions and their variety and distribution. Uncertainty prevails as to the natural history of the processes connecting the lipid lesions with the fissuring plaques, and very little is known about underlying mechanisms. The remaining comments can, therefore, do no more than make selected references to some recent evidence.

There is no doubt that, in the formation of lipid lesions, the major rate-determining factor is the concentration of LDL in plasma. Recent results of studies by S. Shafi, N. J. Cusack and myself indicate that the uptake of LDL by arteries is also accelerated by plasma noradrenaline. This observation may explain, at least in part, the status of coronary risk factors, such as cigarette-smoking, associated with plasma noradrenaline. Other influences on lipid lesion formation may yet be discovered.

It is controversial whether or not a proportion of lipid lesions progresses towards fibrous plaques. Such plaques may become calcified but, again, the mechanism(s) is not yet clear. However, on the basis of experimental work by A. Fleckenstein and G. Fleckenstein-Grün, who discovered the calcium antagonists, a recent clinical trial has provided evidence that prolonged administration of one such agent, nifedipine, significantly decreased the appearance of new lesions demonstrable angiographically in the coronary arteries. If confirmed, this result implies that calcium contributes significantly to the progress of coronary heart disease and that it may be possible to hinder its progress therapeutically. Again, the mechanism underlying this important conclusion is far from clear.

Finally, increasing evidence indicates that macrophages are involved in several stages of the disease process: as lipid-laden 'foam cells'; as sources of cellular growth factors; and of connective tissue-destroying enzymes whereby, according to recent results of studies by C. Lendon, M. J. Davies, P. D. Richardson and myself, these cells may be responsible for weakening plaque caps and so render them liable to fissuring.

The addition of this authoritative volume to the vast body of literature on atherosclerosis is fully justified by the persistent preeminence of the disease.

Gustav V R Born
London, 1990

The William Harvey Research Institute,
St. Bartholomew's Hospital Medical College,
Charterhouse Square, London

CONTENTS

1

Atherosclerosis and its Genesis

Atherosclerosis has existed as a named entity for less than a century (1). It is, however, a pathological process of very considerable antiquity (Figure 1.1); changes consistent with atherosclerosis have been found in mummies of the Eighteenth Dynasty of the pharaohs of Egypt, including that of Merneptah (reigning 1224-1214 BC), who has been traditionally regarded as the pharaoh of the Exodus (2-4). Despite this long history, well reviewed by Morgan (5) and Long (6), our understanding of many of the fundamental aspects of the genesis and progression of atherosclerosis is still far from complete. Until relatively recently, therefore, atherosclerosis has been defined mainly in the context of morphology. While this approach has clear limitations in terms of our understanding of mechanisms, it nevertheless constitutes both a foundation and stimulus for the studies made possible by modern methodology.

At a symposium at the Royal Society of Medicine in 1960, Sir Theo Crawford (7) defined atherosclerosis as:

Figure 1.1
Depiction by Cruveilhier (1827) of the salient features of atherosclerosis: Predilection for large elastic and muscular arteries; focal distribution of the lesions; characteristic intimal thickening.

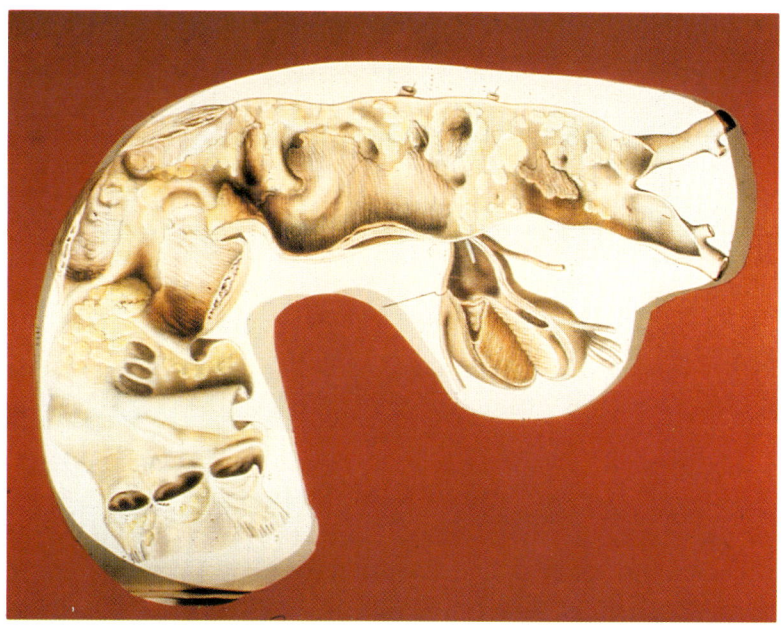

"... the widely prevalent arterial lesion characterized by patchy thickening of the intima, the thickenings comprising accumulations of fat and layers of collagen-like fibres, both being present in widely varying proportions."

This definition, while couched exclusively in morphological terms, nevertheless emphasizes important aspects of the pathology of atherosclerosis which relate to its genesis and natural history (see Box).

Atherosclerotic plaques have a focal distribution which is almost certainly governed by haemodynamic factors.

The intima, rather than the deeper layers of the arterial wall, is predominantly, though not exclusively, involved.

Atherosclerotic lesions are complex, consisting of lipid, most of which is derived from plasma, necrotic connective tissue at the plaque bases and a layer of fibromuscular tissue, forming a covering or 'cap' which separates the other plaque constituents from the blood flowing in the arterial lumen.

Figure 1.2
Diagrammatic representation of normal (left) and atherosclerotic (right) artery wall anatomy to show the three major processes in atherogenesis.

Use of these morphological features as a basis from which to infer the biological mechanisms of plaque genesis, growth and complications may result in three conclusions (Figure 1.2; see Box).

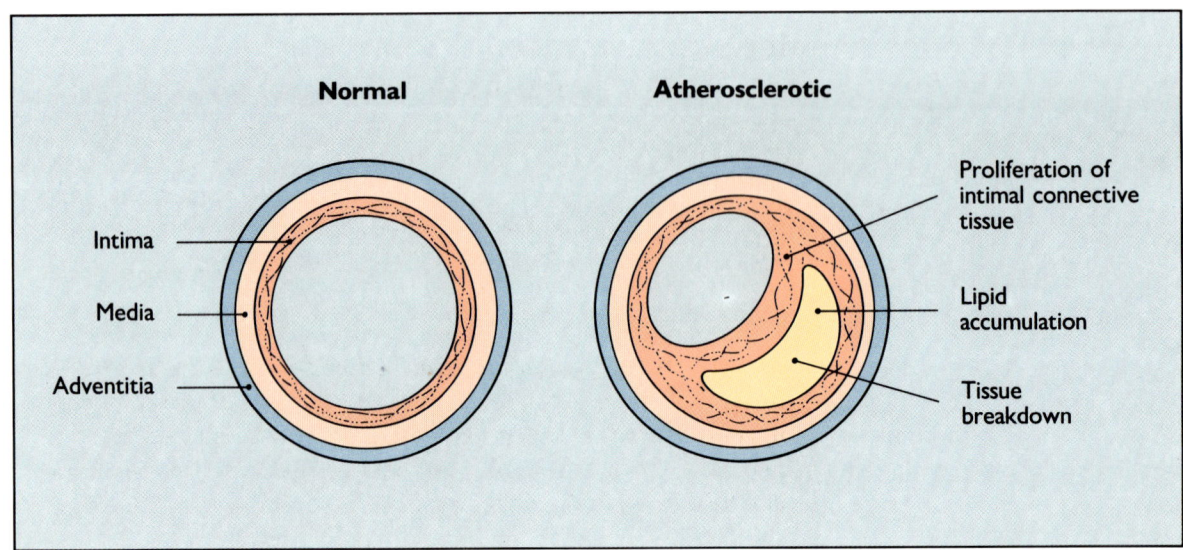

> **Atherosclerosis may be the result of:**
>
> Excess infiltration and/or retention of plasma-derived lipid within the arterial intima;
>
> Connective tissue proliferation, resulting in the formation of the fibromuscular cap mentioned above;
>
> Necrosis of connective tissue at the plaque base, leading to the formation of a 'soft' plaque with a thin cap which, presumably, may rupture readily.

The functional result of intimal fibromuscular proliferation is narrowing of the arterial lumen as seen in the coronary arteries of patients with stable angina. Plaque necrosis, on the other hand, if severe, is likely to be associated with potentially crippling or life-threatening clinical situations such as unstable angina, myocardial infarction or sudden death. All of these are the result of the acute intraplaque and intraluminal thrombosis following fracture of the connective tissue cap of the lesion which allows blood to flow rapidly into the substance of the plaque and, thus, become exposed to thrombogenic components of the arterial wall which are normally shielded by the intact endothelial lining (8-10). The possible mechanisms underlying these events will be discussed after consideration of the basic morphological spectrum of atherosclerotic lesions occuring 'spontaneously' in humans, and as a result of dietary and other manipulations in animal models.

Morphology of atherosclerotic lesions

The logical approach to the question of the morphology and pathogenesis of atherosclerotic lesions would be to first describe the earliest lesion, and then the sequence of changes that lead to the mature, clinically significant, plaque and the complications to which it is heir. However, such a sequential description cannot be given; as Haust (11) has stated,

> *"There is controversy as to what constitutes the earliest lesion, no certainty that the common end-point – the raised fibrolipid plaque – may not be reached from different beginnings and, certainly, no agreement that what, almost by convention, are called 'early atherosclerotic lesions' develop inevitably into characteristic plaques."*

This is particularly *à propos* in relation to the last of her propositions, as the histopathologist must, perforce, view any lesion at only one moment in its natural history. A description of the events that led up to that point and of those likely to follow can only be the result of imaginative reconstruction.

In a number of animal models, one of the earliest structural changes reported is the adhesion of monocytes to the endothelial surface and their subsequent entry into the subendothelial tissue, where they ingest large quantities of lipid and possibly modulate a number of events significant in the development of lesions (12-15). In one model (the White Carneau pigeon, which has a marked diet-independent susceptibility to develop atherosclerosis), monocyte adhesion is associated with an increase in endothelial cell turnover, manifested by a greater than normal incorporation of ^{3}H-thymidine into these cells (16). Although there is sound morphological evidence suggesting that there is monocyte traffic between the blood and arterial wall in atherosclerotic lesions in man, sound data as to the sequence of events in man are much more difficult to obtain than in other animal species. Thus, many pathologists prefer to begin their analysis of the events in atherogenesis from the study of morphologically recognizable lesions.

Fatty streaks

The fatty streak can be seen in large elastic and muscular arteries, such as the aorta and the coronary arteries, from childhood onwards, as observed in vessels *post mortem* from a wide variety of both races and geographical locations. This is in marked contrast to the prevalence of fully developed atherosclerosis which shows considerable geographical variation. This epidemiological difference between the two types of lesion is still a challenging problem.

The extent of intimal surface involvement and the distribution pattern of fatty streaks can be determined by naked-eye examination, made easier if the vessel is stained with a fat-soluble dye such as oil red-0, or a mixture of Sudan dyes. The lesions appear to develop from small (1 to 2 mm diameter) rounded or oval yellowish dots slightly raised above the surface of the adjacent intima. These dots tend to arise in rows lying more or less parallel to the direction of blood flow and coalesce to form streaks along the long axes of the affected artery. Fatty streaks in the aorta are seen in more than 40% of infants coming to necropsy between the ages of one month and one year (17). In the youngest children, the lesions are localized to the region of the aortic valve ring, the area of the ductus scar and the ostia of the intercostal vessels. As the child grows, the aortic arch and the posterior wall of the thoracic aorta become more severely affected, and streak lesions may appear in the abdominal aorta. In the coronary artery tree, well-defined fatty streaks appear in the proximal segments of the vessels at about the time of puberty.

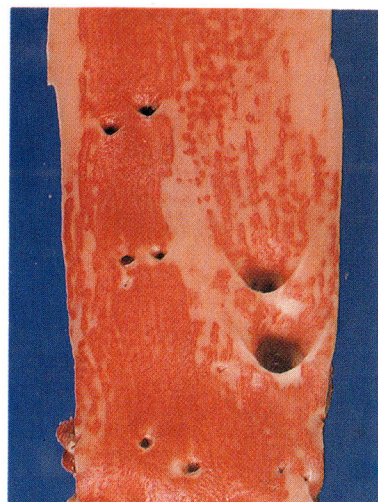

Figure 1.3
Aorta of a young male stained with a fat-soluble dye which shows lipid deposition as red fatty dots and streaks. Note the predilection for the proximal part of the ostia of the branches, and the relative sparing of the flow divider.

Pattern of distribution

In young people, fatty streaks tend to be concentrated in the arch and upper part of the ascending aorta in a fan-shaped distribution. From a point 5 to 7 cm distal to its most proximal portion, the 'fan' narrows and the streaks become most obvious on the posterior wall of the aorta. Distal to the main visceral aortic branches, the distribution pattern changes and the entire circumference of the aorta becomes apparently haphazardly involved. In the thoracic aorta of young people, the streak lesions are most apparent in the proximal portions of the intercostal vessel ostia, and there is relative sparing of the distal edges or 'flow-divider' regions of the ostia (Figure 1.3). A similar pattern in relation to intercostal arteries is seen in hyperlipidaemic animal species, provided that the cholesterol concentrations in blood and tissues are in steady-state (18-20). Thus, there appears to be a predilection for lipid deposition and, hence, streak lesion formation where the arterial wall shear rates (the velocity gradients between layers of fluid in contact with and near to the arterial wall) are low, and where non-atherosclerotic intimal thickening is much greater than in the flow-divider regions, where the wall shear rate is high (Figures 1.4 & 1.5).

Histological examination of the fatty streak shows localized thickening of the intima associated with the presence of fat droplets, easily seen in frozen sections stained with fat-soluble dyes. The fat appears to be predominantly intracellularly localized although, in some lesions, there is a sprinkling of sudanophilic material along the course of the internal elastic lamina which marks the boundary between the intima and the media.

Cell population of the streak lesion
Although the cell population of the streak is much larger than in the uninvolved intima, the nature of the cells is not dis-

Figure 1.4
Histological section of a branch point in the aorta of a young female. The direction of blood flow is from right to left and the flow divider is to the left. Note the focal intimal thickening at the proximal part of the ostium, where the wall shear rate is low.

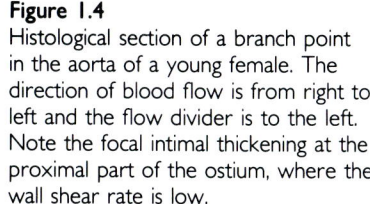

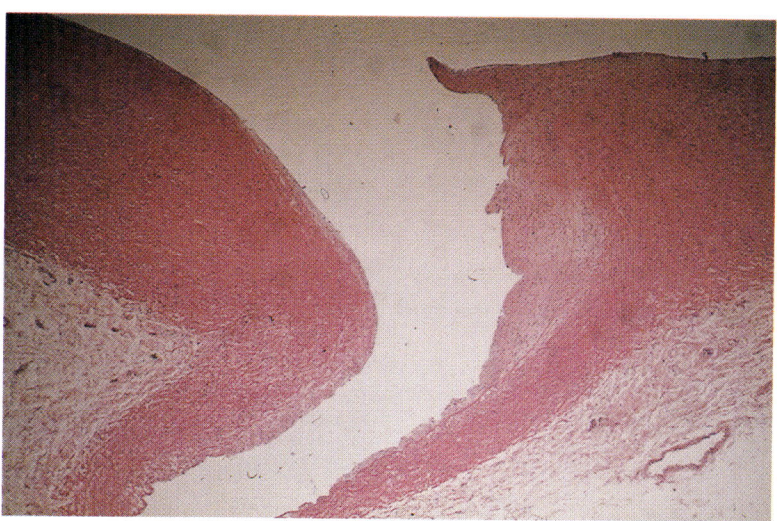

Figure 1.5
Diagrammatic representation of lipid depositions in relation to blood flow and vessel branching.

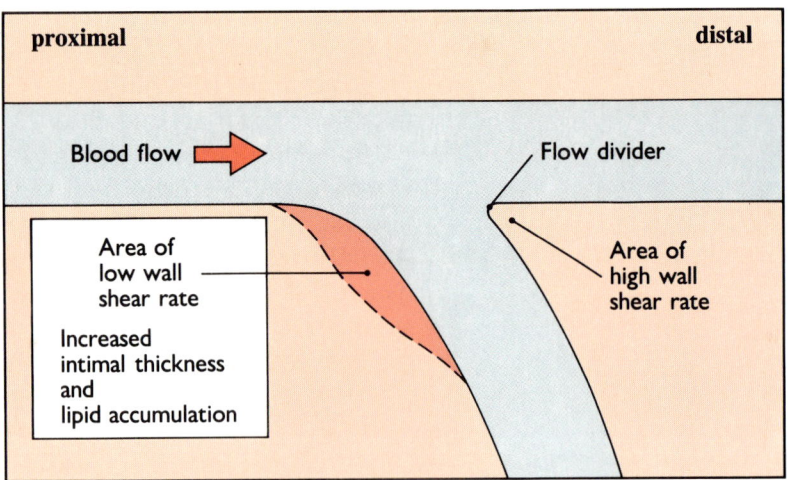

cernible on light microscopy without use of the appropriate immunohistochemical methods. A significant proportion of the cells are derived from monocytes and show macrophage markers (21-24). This observation is supported by electronmicroscopic examination of fatty streaks (see Box).

> At least two cell types can be identified:
>
> One is an intimal smooth muscle cell identifiable by its elongated profile, the presence of 'dense bodies' (the analogue of Z bands) at the cell periphery and the evidence of basal lamina formation. A few lipid vacuoles are also seen in this cell type.
> The second cell type lacks an elongated profile, and has a ruffled and convoluted plasma membrane.
> The cytoplasm contains numerous lipid vacuoles and occasional 'myelin figures', features suggesting that this segment of the cell population consists of macrophages.

Despite these characteristics, it must be remembered that, once a cell becomes heavily loaded with lipid, identification based on morphology may become impossible and immunohistochemical staining of appropriate differentiation markers may be necessary. Identification of the macrophage as a significant element in the cell population of fatty streaks and, indeed, of mature atherosclerotic lesions is an important advance towards a more complete understanding of the mechanisms involved in atherogenesis as the macrophage may exercise a range of functions within the arterial intima far beyond its conventional role in phagocytosis.

As transmission electron microscopy has increased our knowledge of the cell population of the fatty streak, so has scanning electron microscopy (SEM) increased our appreciation of events taking place at the blood/vessel wall interface during lesion formation and progression. In young hyperlipidaemic rabbits, SEM shows localized areas of subendothelial swelling, which are particularly prominent in the intima immediately upstream of the intercostal artery ostia where, as already stated, wall shear rates are low. Longer periods of hyperlipidaemia are associated with the appearances of focal defects in the integrity of the endothelial lining. These defects are associated with the presence of large cells with markedly ruffled plasma membranes, appearances suggestive of macrophages (Figure 1.6). Not infrequently, individual macrophages can be seen to penetrate between individual endothelial cells and, in some areas, groups of such macrophages can be seen protruding into the arterial lumen from beneath 'bridges' of intact endothelial cells (15). When human coronary arteries are examined by SEM, fatty streak precursors can be seen as small plateau-like subendothelial elevations, some in association with adherent leucocytes (25).

Fate of the fatty streak
Controversy still clouds the issue of whether or not fatty streaks progress to mature fibrolipid atherosclerotic lesions (26). Certainly, not all fatty streaks do so, as the extent of intimal surface involvement by fatty streaks, as seen at necropsy in young subjects, shows no significant differences between populations with a high incidence of severe atherosclerosis and those in which extensive and severe atherosclerosis is not seen. Histological examination of lesions in man shows an intermediate-type lesion which suggests that progression from a fatty streak to a fibrolipid lesion may occur. In addition,

Figure 1.6
Scanning electron micrograph (EM) from a lesion-free area of the aorta from a hyperlipidaemic rabbit. Adhering to the endothelial surface is a white cell showing the typical 'ruffled' plasma membrane of a monocyte/macrophage.

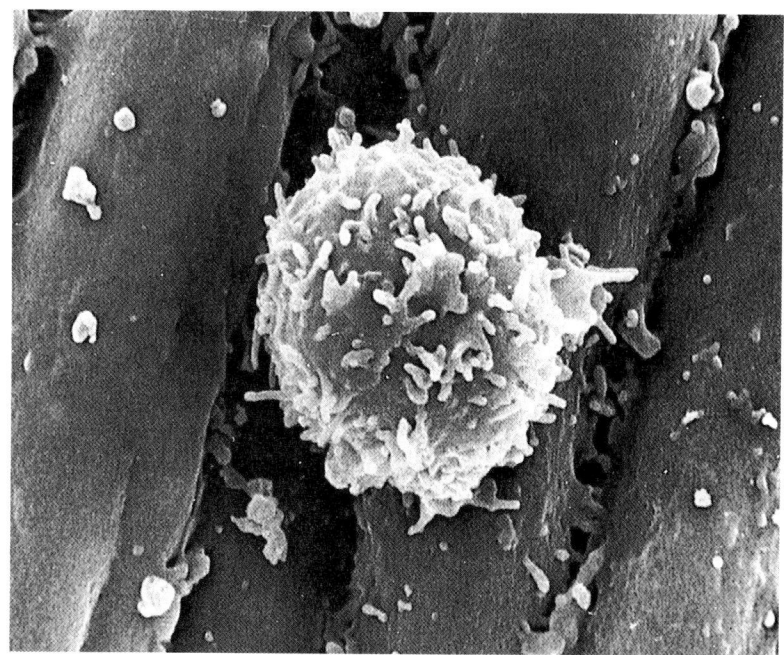

a recent study by Faggiotto and Ross (27) on the long-term effects of diet-related hyperlipidaemia on the arteries of primates provides persuasive supporting morphological evidence. This combination of morphological and epidemiological data suggests that some fatty streaks which originate early in life undergo regression while others grow into mature atherosclerotic plaques (Figure 1.7). The latter are, presumably, more likely to occur in populations with a greater degree of risk factors for atherogenesis, such as hyperlipidaemia, cigarette-smoking, high blood pressure and diabetes mellitus. At the fatty-streak stage, it is very difficult, if not impossible, to distinguish between those lesions likely to progress and those which will not. In an histological study carried out on fatty streaks *post mortem* from young subjects from several populations showing the greatest discordance between the degree of fatty streaks in the young and the degree of involvement by fibrolipid plaques in the middle-aged and elderly, Restrepo and Tracy (28) equated the presence of focal necrosis and a severe inflammatory cell infiltrate within the lesion with the likelihood of progression.

Gelatinous lesions

Wolkoff (29) was the first to suggest that small blister-like elevations in the arterial intima may be the precursors of mature atherosclerotic plaques. These translucent droplet-like lesions are more difficult to see than the opaque fatty streaks and therefore may have been overlooked in post-mortem surveys. Indeed, there is no recent data of their prevalence and topographical distribution within the arterial tree (30).

Most of the available descriptions of gelatinous elevations record their presence in all parts of the aorta. They are small,

Figure 1.7
Possible fates of the fatty streak.

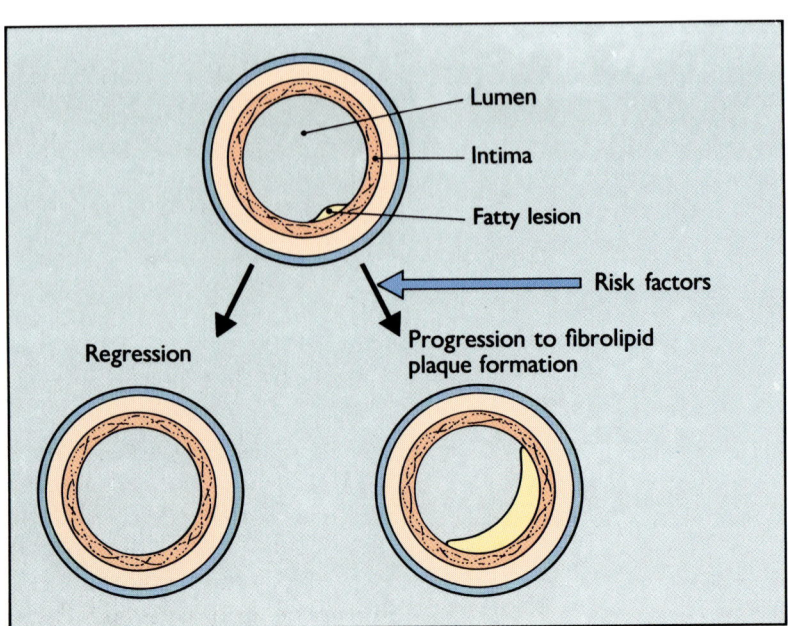

oval or, sometimes, streak-like, and are most often colourless or a very pale pink, though occasionally a yellowish tinge may be noted.

The histological appearances of the gelatinous elevation are extremely banal, consisting essentially of separation of the formed elements of connective tissue by interstitial oedema. Intimal smooth muscle cells appear to be predominant. Stainable fat is present usually only in small amounts and tends to be distributed diffusely through the intima. There is an increased local concentration of certain plasma proteins, notably fibrinogen and low-density lipoprotein (LDL) in a concentration four times greater than that of normal intima, and albumin, but to a lesser extent (30). Staining by both conventional methods and immunohistochemistry shows the presence of finely dispersed fibrin or fibrinogen within the slightly thickened intima (31-33). After extraction of soluble fibrinogen from these lesions, controlled incubation of the residual tissue with plasmin produces a nearly fifteen-fold greater release of fibrin degradation products (FDP) than does normal intima (34). These FDP contain a high proportion of D-dimer characteristic of cross-linked fibrin, and Smith suggests that this is consistent with fibrin deposition playing a significant part in the development of this lesion. FDP are chemotactic for monocytes (35) and stimulate mitogenesis (36). Extracts of gelatinous lesions stimulate DNA synthesis in the chick chorioallantoic membrane and it is suggested that this activity resides within the FDP fraction (36).

These data support the view that the gelatinous elevation is a form of focal intimal oedema (11). Whether it is the precursor lesion for fully developed atherosclerotic plaques is as yet uncertain. Questions yet to be answered in the evaluation of this problem relate to their distribution and frequency (see Box).

Do gelatinous elevations occur at sites of predilection for mature atherosclerotic plaques?

Do they occur in greater numbers in populations which later present with more severe and extensive atherosclerosis?

Raised lesions (fibrolipid plaques)
The raised lesion or fibrolipid plaque is the archetypal lesion of atherosclerosis, and complications of this lesion, notably plaque fissure or ulceration, are the basis of the vast majority of cases of occlusive arterial disease. Unlike the fatty streak, the extent of intimal involvement by fibrolipid plaques appears to predict the frequency and severity of the clinical manifestations of atherosclerosis in given populations (37-39). In the

aorta, these plaques are seen most frequently in the abdominal portions of the vessel and often involve the mouths of intercostal and lumbar arteries. In vessels such as the common carotid artery, rarely are lesions more advanced than fatty streaks found, although calcified and ulcerated fibrolipid plaques are commonly seen in the region just beyond the bifurcation of the common carotid artery. This modulation of the natural history of atherosclerotic lesions is presumably mediated by haemodynamic factors.

All fibrolipid plaques share two basic morphological components: A connective tissue cap, which lies immediately beneath the endothelium; and an underlying 'atheromatous pool' of lipid-rich, mostly necrotic debris. Within these limits there are many morphological variants, most of which are the expression of differences in the relative proportions of the cap and the atheromatous pool, and the sequelae of such differences (Figures 1.8 & 1.9).

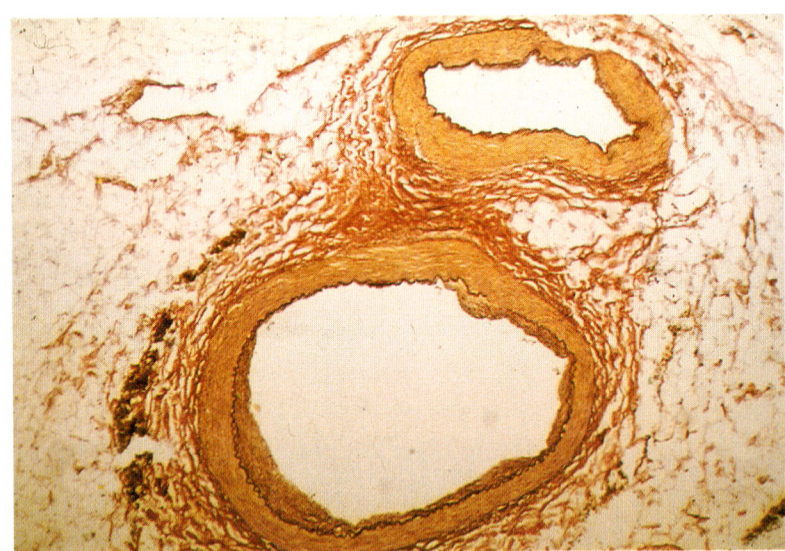

Figure 1.8
Histological transverse section through the coronary arteries of a young child stained (black) to show the internal elastic lamina marking the boundary between the intima and the media. Note the thin delicate intima characteristic at this phase of life.

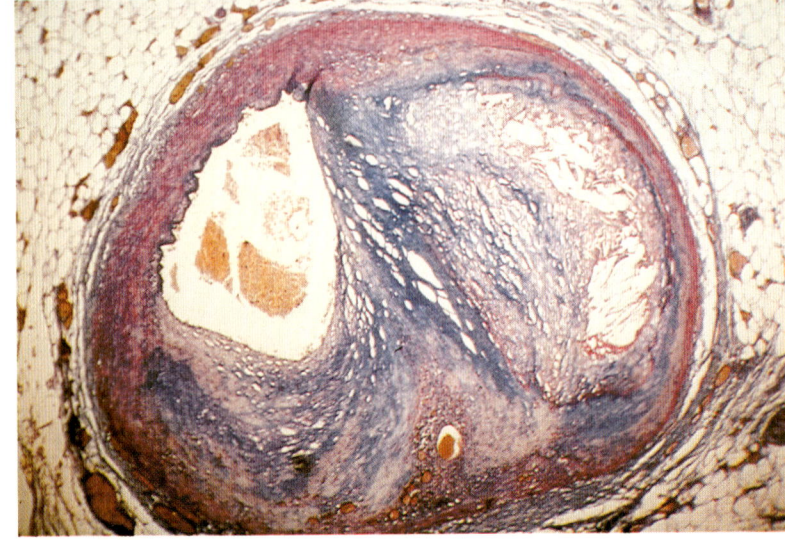

Figure 1.9
Histological transverse section through the coronary artery of a male in late middle age. The cross-sectional luminal area is reduced by approximately 70% due to a large, eccentric atheromatous plaque. As trichrome staining shows collagen as blue, it is obvious that the major contributor to vessel narrowing in this case is connective tissue proliferation.

Fibrolipid plaques are considerably raised above the surface of the surrounding non-involved intima. The media underlying the plaques often shows a significant degree of secondary thinning but, even in its absence, the thickness of the plaque intima may exceed that of the media and adventitia combined. In some lesions, the proliferated connective tissue cap is the predominant element, conferring an opaque pearl-like appearance to the plaque. In cross-section, the yellow lipid-rich base may be inconspicuous or absent (Figure 1.10). These firm plaques may cause luminal narrowing, but are seldom associated with rupture or acute intralesional or intraluminal thrombosis. In a study of advanced fibrous plaques within the femoral artery, the caps were found to consist of dense connective tissue with spaces infilled with pancake-shaped cells showing characteristics of smooth muscle cells. Electron microscopy revealed that these smooth muscle cell-containing lacunae consisted of concentrically arranged layers of basement membrane, collagen fibres and proteoglycans (40).

In other lesions, the basal accumulation of lipid, tissue debris and other blood-derived constituents may be of such massive proportions that this 'pool' is separated from the lumen only by a thin, easily ruptured sheet of fibromuscular tissue (Figure 1.11). It is this type of plaque which is particularly at risk of major thrombotic events and suggests that basal necrosis within the plaque may be a key factor in the genesis of occlusive atherosclerosis-related disease. The pathological changes in fibrolipid plaques and their sequelae are described in Chapter 2.

Figure 1.10
Histological transverse section through the coronary artery showing a large plaque composed almost exclusively of fibromuscular connective tissue.

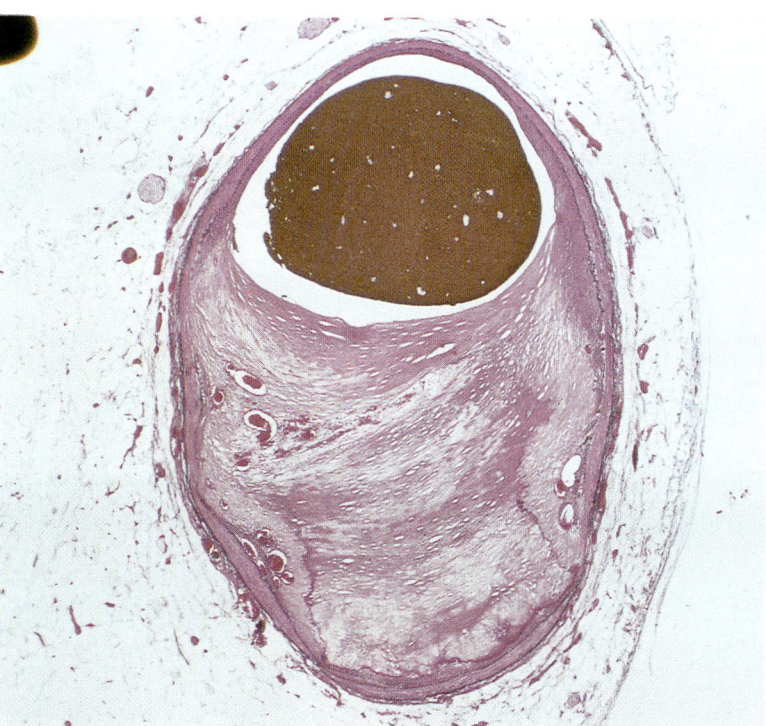

Figure 1.11
Histological transverse section
through a coronary artery showing
concentric narrowing of the lumen by
atherosclerosis. The plaque contains
a massive basal pool which is rich in
lipid and probably deficient in collagen.
The pool is separated from the lumen
(containing radiopaque material) by a
thin connective tissue 'cap'.

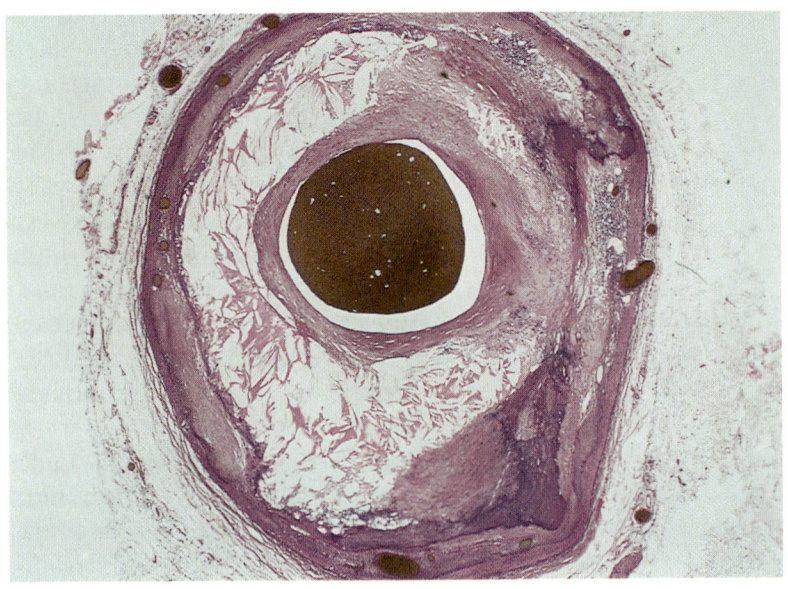

Fibrolipid plaque-related medial changes
A considerable degree of medial thinning often occurs beneath
fibrolipid plaques, the extent and severity of which may contribute to whether stenosis is 'fixed' or variable. These medial changes may reflect disturbances in nutrition of the arterial wall. The adventitia and outer two-thirds of the media are
supplied by diffusion from the vasa vasorum of the superficial
adventitia, while the intima and the inner third of the media
are nourished by diffusion from blood in the vessel lumen. The
interface between these two zones is most likely to suffer from
disturbances of nutrition. A significant degree of intimal thickening, for example, will prevent lumen-derived nutrients from
reaching the requisite depth within the vessel wall. These concepts have received some support from histochemical studies
showing that, with increasing age and increasing intimal thickness, the mid-zone of the media is the site of reduced respira-
tory enzyme activity (41).

Fibrolipid plaque-related adventitial changes
Fibrolipid plaques may be associated with three changes in the
surrounding adventitia (41; see Box).

An increase in fibrous tissue;

An increase in vascularity;

The frequent presence of cellular aggregates consisting
primarily of B-lymphocytes.

Adventitial lymphocytic aggregates were first described in the English literature as long ago as 1915 (43). The most extensive and systematic study of this phenomenon was carried out by Schwartz and Mitchell (44). Their findings indicated that the major determinant for this feature was plaque severity and that it was generally independent of age, gender and site within the arterial tree. The intensity of adventitial cellularity was also found to be related to the presence within the affected segments of recent thrombosis. Recent attempts to explain these appearances have focused on the likelihood that such lymphocytic infiltrates are the expression of an immune response to oxidized lipids and ceroid in intralesional macrophages (45).

Fibrolipid plaque-related mural thrombosis
Mural thrombi arise not infrequently in relation to established fibrolipid plaques and may become incorporated into the substance of the artery wall (Figure 1.12). The degree of local intimal thickening may then be increased, in part by the bulk of unorganized residuum of the thrombus and partly because of the platelet-driven proliferative response. Much of the comparatively recent interest in the putative role of mural thrombosis as a contributor to plaque growth stems from the studies of the late J. B. Duguid (46-48), who put forward the view that many of the lesions classified as atherosclerotic are, in fact, altered thrombi which, by the process of organization, have been transformed into fibrous intimal thickenings. Duguid suggested that this represents a partial return to the encrustation hypothesis advanced by Rokitansky a century earlier (49).

Figure 1.12
Histological section of an aortic atherosclerotic plaque showing the presence of mural thrombus. Trichrome staining shows fibrin as red and platelets as grey-blue. Part of the plaque cap consists entirely of recent thrombus and, deep to this and separated by a band of connective tissue, is similarly staining material, the remains of a previously incorporated mural thrombus.

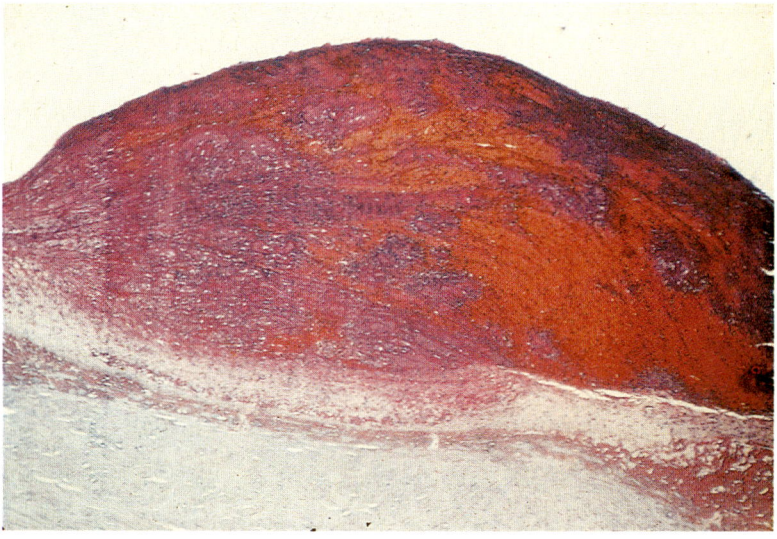

In many cases, it is easy to differentiate between mural thrombi and subendothelial deposits or the remains of previously incorporated thrombotic material on histological examination (5,47,50). Crawford and Levene (51), in a study of lesion-free aortas showing slight roughening, found that of 99 roughened areas, 19 had surface encrustations, 10 had superficial but subendothelial deposits, and 24 showed material with the staining properties of fibrin lying deep within the intima.

Figure 1.13
Histological section of the connective tissue cap of an aortic plaque treated with a fluorescein-linked anti-human platelet serum. The sites of antibody binding appear as bands of fluorescent material within the thickened intima, indicating incorporated mural thrombus.

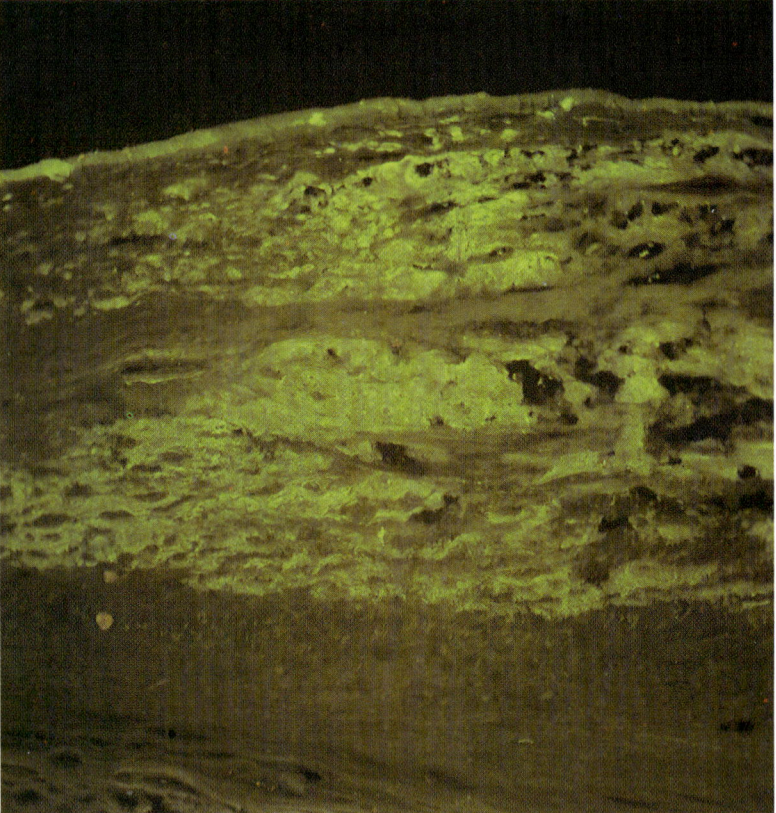

The presence of fibrin can be demonstrated more sensitively and reliably by the use of immunohistochemistry. Fibrinogen and fibrin are present in many atherosclerotic lesions (52). By examining the different morphological patterns of binding of antibodies raised against human fibrin, it may be possible to determine whether fibrin or fibrinogen is present as a result of insudation or as a marker of incorporated mural thrombus (33). This has been confirmed by immunohistology (53-55) and other methods (56). Although the presence of fibrin either on or within the arterial intima does not, in itself, indicate mural thrombosis, it is not likely that aggregates of platelets occur within the vessel wall because of another process. Carstairs (57) was the first to identify platelet masses within atherosclerotic lesions using immunofluorescence. Subsequent studies (58,59) have shown that platelet antigens are found only in raised lesions and not in fatty streaks, and that their presence correlates with a pattern of antifibrin binding suggestive of incorporation of thrombus (Figure 1.13). Such residua of thrombi may be found in up to 90% of plaques in a single aorta and in up to 33% of coronary lesions (60). There is apparently little doubt, therefore, that incorporation of mural thrombi frequently occurs in relation to established atherosclerotic plaques. Indeed, it is not unlikely that this frequency may have been underestimated (58).

A significant positive correlation between these aortic plaques with immunohistological appearances suggestive of incorporated thrombus and the presence of ischaemic heart disease has been found (61). Whether this reflects an increased tendency to arterial thrombosis is not certain, but it is consistent with epidemiological evidence that raised plasma fibrinogen and factor VII concentrations constitute independent risk factors for coronary heart disease (CHD) (62,63).

Major atherogenic processes in man and other animals

Connective tissue proliferation and arterial smooth muscle cells

When a plaque encroaches on the integrity of a vessel lumen, it does so by a striking focal increase in the amount of intimal connective tissue. The cell type essential to this process is the intimal smooth muscle cell, which is seen in the 'normal' arterial intima of young animals, in areas of either diffuse or focal intimal thickening, the latter often at points of branching in the coronary arteries of infants, and in atherosclerotic lesions.

The intimal population of smooth muscle cells is thought to be derived from the migration of medial smooth muscle cells through fenestrae in the internal elastic lamina, although the intimal cells show distinct phenotypic differences from their medial counterparts. Within the intima, smooth muscle cells are elongated and show basal lamina formation. In normal intima, the cells show fewer contractile filaments than do fully differentiated medial smooth muscle cells, and there is a similar decrease in the number of peripheral 'dense bodies', the analogues of Z bands, compared with medial smooth muscle. Of the many characteristics of arterial smooth muscle cells, perhaps the most interesting is their ability to present more than one phenotypic form. At one extreme is a smooth muscle cell which functions almost entirely as a contractile cell; at the other extreme is a cell which is almost exclusively concerned with proliferation and synthesis of a number of extracellular tissue components (Figure 1.14).

The expression of the various phenotypes is controlled by the interaction of a series of chemical signals, which may exert their effect either by directly stimulating smooth muscle

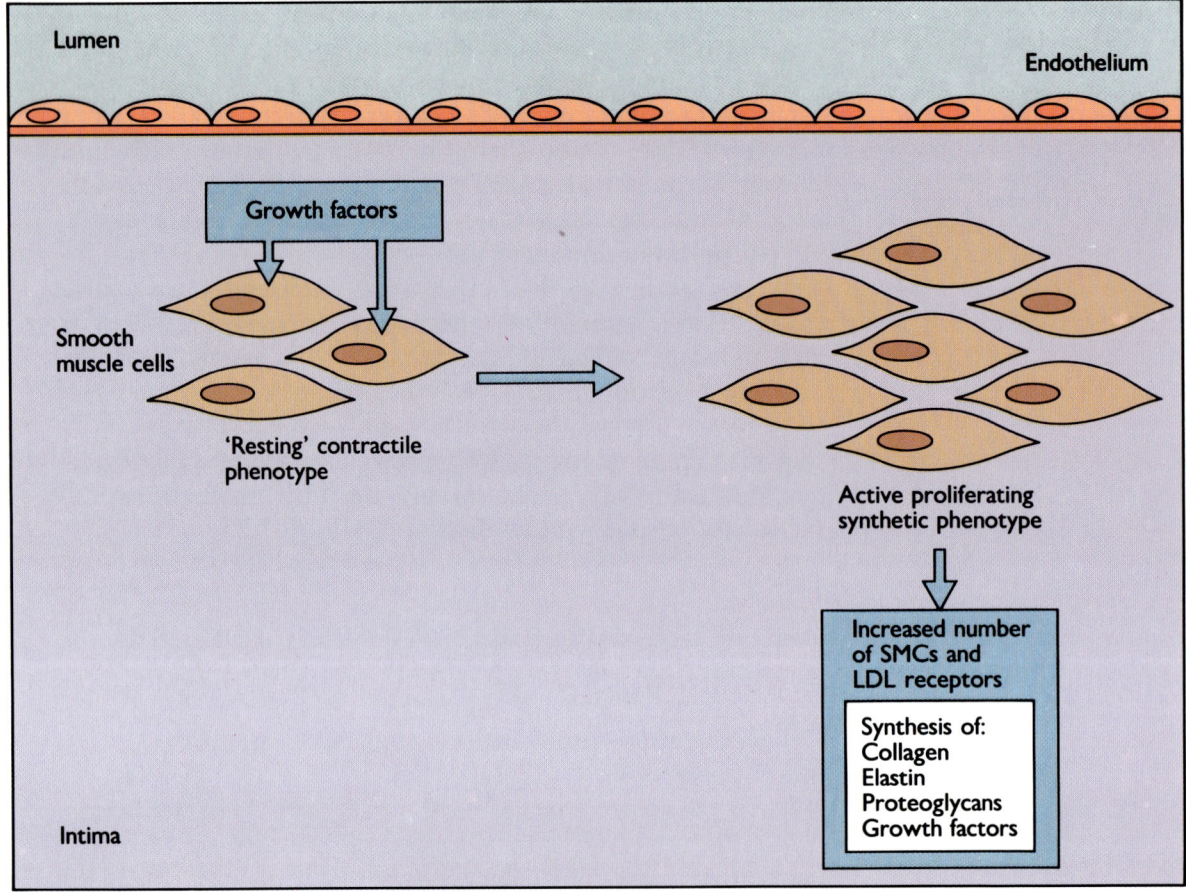

Figure 1.14
Diagram showing two functionally distinct phenotypes that can be manifested by intimal smooth muscle cells.

cells through a receptor-ligand interaction, or by removal of a particular inhibitory influence(s). In the non-contractile phenotype, these cells possess the ability to proliferate to a striking degree in response to local increases in growth factors, which may be *via* paracrine release from nearby endothelial cells (see Figure 1.23), platelets or macrophages, or autocrine release from the smooth muscle cells themselves.

The behaviour of these cells has been studied in a number of models of arterial injury followed by migration and proliferation of medial smooth muscle cells within the intima (Figures 1.15 – 1.17). The resulting neointima may be many times as thick as non-injured adjacent intima. During the stage of active proliferation, the new smooth muscle cells show considerable morphological as well as chemical differences from mature medial smooth muscle cells, as they contain decreased amounts of actin and desmin, and increased amounts of vimentin. Within 10 to 11 weeks, however, when the damaged arterial endothelium has regenerated completely, the cytoskeleton of the new intimal smooth muscle cells has become similar to those of the media (64).

Other features of the altered smooth muscle cell include the expression of plasma membrane receptors for LDL and the ability to secrete a number of prostanoids. The source of the

Figure 1.15
Histological section of aorta from a nine-month-old pig ten days after intimal abrasion. The resulting thrombus appears as an amorphous pink-staining material covered by layers of proliferating smooth muscle cells in response to local release of growth factors.

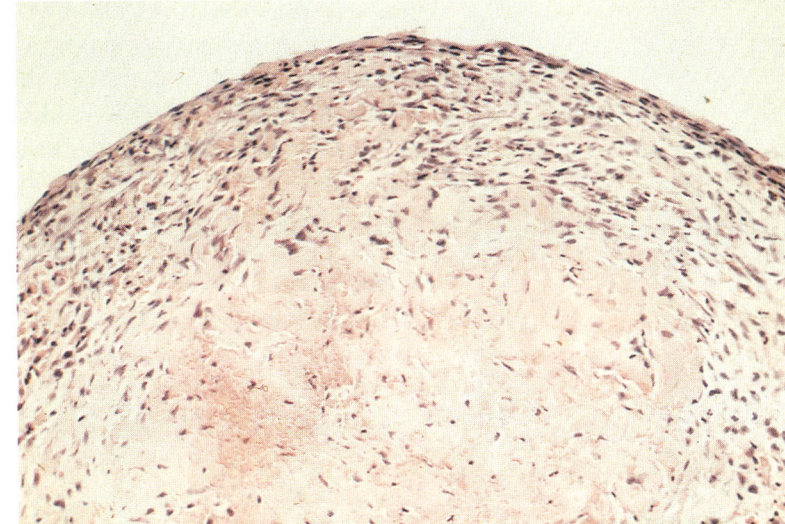

Figure 1.16
Histological section of aorta from a nine-month-old pig three weeks after intimal abrasion. There is a grossly thickened neointima showing numerous red-staining smooth muscle cells.

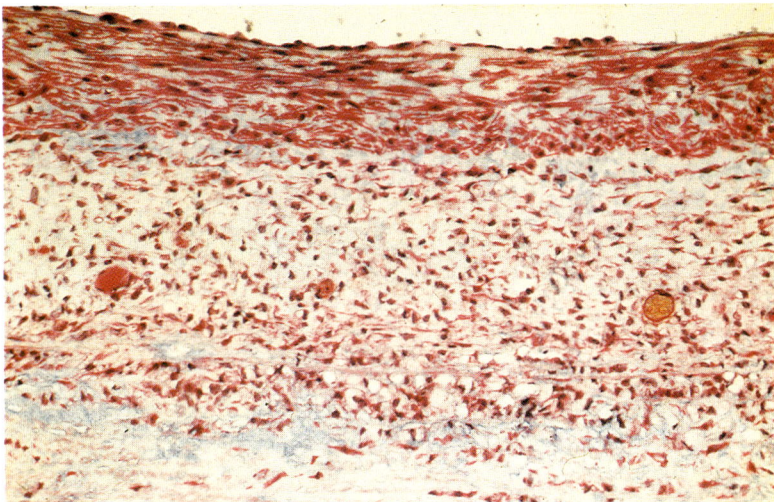

Figure 1.17
Histological section of aorta from a rabbit, fed a diet containing 1% cholesterol, at five weeks after balloon-catheter injury. Note the localized plaque-like intimal thickening showing a considerable degree of lipid deposition (stained red).

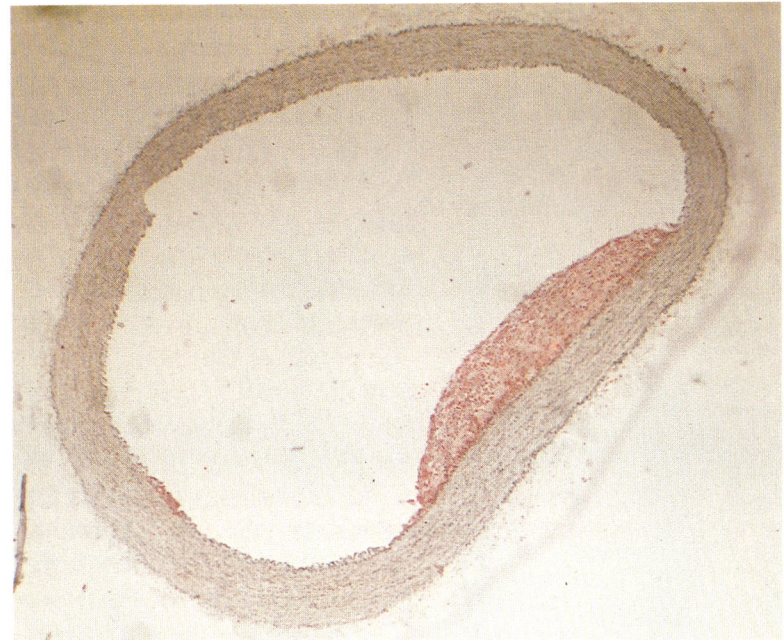

new extracellular connective tissue formed both in the course
of atherogenesis and in response to arterial injury is almost certainly the smooth muscle cell in its synthetic phenotype (65).
There is compelling evidence that medial smooth muscle cells
derived by explant culture from primate aortas produce not
only soluble elastin, but large amounts of a glycoprotein with
an amino-acid composition identical to that found in the mi-
crofibrillar component of intact elastic fibres (66,67). Ross (68)
found that cultured arterial smooth muscle cells secrete collagen and this was confirmed by McCullagh and Balian (69).
Arterial smooth muscle cells in culture also show the ability
to produce glycosaminoglycans, the most quantitatively prominent being dermatan sulphate. As a major portion of the connective tissue cap of a fibrolipid plaque consists of these very
components, these ex-vivo findings may be highly significant
(see Box).

> A reasonable assumption may be that modulation of
> the arterial smooth muscle cells from the **contractile**
> to the **synthetic** phenotype is responsible for the
> connective tissue proliferation which is a key element
> in the evolution of atherosclerosis.

The role of growth factors in controlling the intimal smooth muscle cell population

Our understanding of the putative mechanisms involved in the
altered phenotypes of arterial smooth muscle cells (see above)
is based on the studies of Ross and colleagues. They showed
that the mitogenic effect of serum derived from whole clotted
blood on arterial smooth muscle cells in culture is primarily
due to a factor released from platelets, so-called 'platelet-derived growth factor' (PDGF) (67,70-75). This term, however,
is a misnomer because, although it is certainly stored in and
released from platelets (together with platelet factor IV and
beta-thromboglobulin), it may also be produced by endothelial cells, macrophages and arterial smooth muscle cells in their
synthetic phenotype. It is a cationic dimeric protein with a
molecular weight of 28,000 to 32,000 which is stored as the
heterodimer in the alpha-granules of platelets. The dimer is
composed of two homologous polypeptide chains, A and B,
and the genes which encode these chains have been mapped
to different chromosomes; thus, their expression is indepen-
dently regulated (76,77).

PDGF binds with high affinity to receptors on arterial
smooth muscle cells, fibroblasts, 3T3 cells (an immortalized
line of murine fibroblasts) and other mesenchymal cells, although there is no evidence of binding to arterial endothelium.
It has one important difference from other growth factors thus

far discovered: It is not only mitogenic but also chemoattractant, which may account for the migration of smooth muscle cells from the media seen in atherogenesis and in response to arterial injury.

> PDGF is a **competence** rather than **progression** type of growth factor: It brings the cells to which it binds out of G_0 and into the cell cycle rather than only affecting cells already in cycle (mitogenic effect).

Binding of PDGF to its receptor causes activation of the phosphatidylinositol pathway, the transcription of c-*myc* and c-*fos* proto-oncogenes and an increase in both cytoplasmic calcium concentration and pH. Its beta chain shows an 87% degree of homology with the gene product of the transforming oncogene of the simian sarcoma virus (v-*sis*) and, more important, with that of the cellular proto-oncogene c-*sis* (78, 79). Expression of this gene is almost certainly an important element in wound repair. The cells of several malignant tumours have been shown to secrete PDGF, which presumably stimulates autocrine proliferation of these cells, as treatment of such cells in culture with antibodies raised against PDGF blocks the incorporation of tritiated thymidine into the tumour cells (80).

Consequences of cellular binding of PDGF
Binding of PDGF to its specific receptor is followed by a series of cellular events, some of which are related to cell division and others to a range of functions apparently unrelated to mitogenesis, such as increased endocytosis, cholesterol synthesis and increased expression of the LDL-receptor. Maximum DNA synthesis occurs in PDGF-stimulated arterial smooth muscle cells in culture within 18 to 24 hours and the cell population doubles within approximately 30 hours. The receptor site, on occupation by the growth factor, acts as a tyrosine kinase and phosphorylates a number of cytoplasmic and plasma membrane-associated proteins. The effect of this protein phosphorylation is not as yet understood, although binding of this growth factor leads to the expression of the nuclear proto-oncogenes c-*myc* and c-*fos*. A significant rise in c-*fos* transcription (50-fold) is initiated within five minutes of treatment of cultured cells with PDGF, and c-*myc* transcription is also activated, although this takes place more slowly. This activation of nuclear proto-oncogenes may be responsible for the cell proliferation caused by PDGF-binding. Transcription of the actin gene is also initiated at approximately 15 minutes from the time of PDGF-binding (Figure 1.18).

In addition to the phosphorylation of tyrosine residues on both the receptor proteins and other specific intracellular pro-

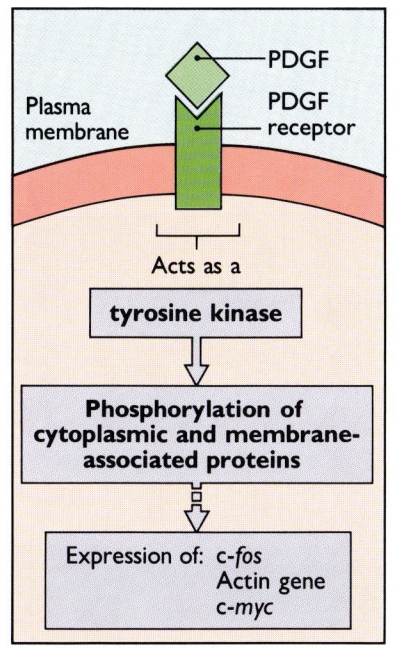

Figure 1.18
Putative pathway of the mitogenic effect of platelet-derived growth factor (PDGF)-binding.

teins, there is also rapid activation of phosphatidylinositol breakdown by phospholipase C, with release of diacylglycerol and inositol-1, 4, 5-triphosphate. Unlike other growth factors [with the exception of fibroblast growth factor (FGF)], PDGF-binding is associated with a massive release of arachidonic acid from the cell, mediated through the activation of phospholipase A_2. Further metabolism of the arachidonic acid may lead to the synthesis of leukotrienes and prostaglandins (81-84).

The generation of IP_3 is thought to mobilize calcium ions from internal pools which, as a consequence, allows the modulation of many calcium-dependent processes (85). The diacylglycerol released as a result of the action of phospholipase C can, perhaps in conjunction with the increase in cytosolic calcium ions, activate protein kinase C which, in turn, may mediate many regulatory processes, for example, the selective alteration in protein synthesis which follows protein kinase C-mediated phosphorylation of ribosomal protein S6. As an essential part of the mitogenic response, protein kinase C also activates the sodium/hydrogen antiport, causing the extrusion of hydrogen ions from the cell and a rapid rise in cellular pH which, together with the rise in cytosolic calcium, is necessary for the transcription of nuclear genes required for DNA synthesis (86; Figure 1.19).

Figure 1.19
Some of the consequences of PDGF – cell interaction.

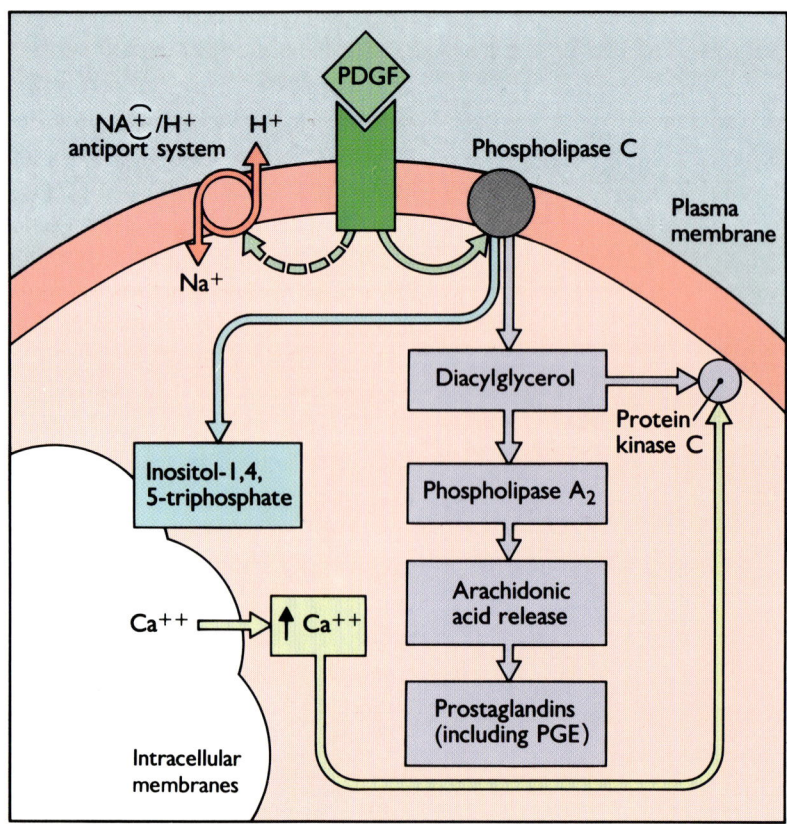

Cellular sources of PDGF

The natural history of lipid-induced atherosclerotic lesions wherein smooth muscle proliferation occurs in the absence of endothelial denudation and platelet adhesion suggests that there are sources other than the platelet of growth factor(s) which are mitogenic for arterial smooth muscle.

Endothelial cells. It has been known for some time that culture media 'conditioned' by endothelial cells are mitogenic for muscle cells in culture (67), and it is now clear that endothelial cells synthesize both the A and B chains of PDGF (87-91). The release of PDGF from endothelium is stimulated by phorbol esters, tumour necrosis factor (TNF) and endotoxin. It has been observed that newly isolated endothelial cells, either from bovine aorta or human umbilical vein, express little messenger RNA (mRNA) for PDGF whereas the same cells in culture show an extremely high level of transcription of the PDGF gene (92); this is important as it suggests that, in cells in culture, the endothelium may be metabolically abnormal (74). It may therefore be unwise to extrapolate too enthusiastically from *in vitro* to *in vivo*.

Smooth muscle cells. Although smooth muscle cells taken from adult rat aorta do not produce significant amounts of PDGF in primary culture, such cells taken from the same vessel in newborn rats do (93). The proliferation of smooth muscle cells is a constant feature of the reaction to balloon-catheter injury in a variety of animal species and has been examined in rats whose carotid arteries were subjected to such an injury. Smooth muscle cells from the injured vessels of these rats were also found to produce PDGF in culture. Once stimulated by PDGF, smooth muscle cells from arteries have been shown to produce an insulin-like growth factor which is a 'progression factor' (mitogenic for cells which are 'in cycle' and not in G_0). When rabbit aortic smooth muscle cells are cultured, the cells in later passages have been found to secrete a mitogenic factor which is apparently distinct from PDGF and has an autocrine effect, stimulating the growth of the smooth muscle cells themselves (94).

Macrophages. A potential growth-promoting role for the macrophage can be inferred from its role in chronic inflammation and wound-healing. When animals are treated with hydrocortisone and an antimacrophage serum, fibroblast proliferation and collagen formation are inhibited (95). Activated macrophages in culture secrete growth factors for smooth muscle, fibroblasts and endothelium (74). The mitogen which these cells secrete was shown to consist of two forms of PDGF (96); these observations have been supported by the demonstration of transcription of the c-*sis* oncogene by activated macrophages

(97). Macrophages also secrete fibroblast growth factor, an effective mitogen for mesenchymal cells (98), transforming growth factor-alpha (99), which binds to the epidermal growth factor-receptor transforming growth factor-beta – a multifunctional peptide with a wide range of unrelated and sometimes apparently conflicting effects on many different types of cell (100,101).

Platelets. In addition to PDGF, platelets secrete other growth factors including EGF (epidermal growth factor) and transforming growth factor-beta (102; Figure 1.20).

Growth factors in atherosclerotic lesions in man
Barrett and Benditt (103) have found elevated levels of mRNA for PDGF in atherosclerotic plaques compared with normal artery wall. They also found that the PDGF-A chain appears to have a similar degree of expression in the smooth muscle cells of both the normal media and in the lesions. Furthermore, Wilcox and colleagues (104), using the techniques of in-situ hybridization, have localized mRNA for both the A and B chains of PDGF to both plaque endothelium and to cells within the intima which they described as 'mesenchymal'. These cells appeared to be transcribing mRNA for the A chain in particular. On microscopy, some of these cells were spindle-shaped and had elongated nuclei, the appearances of smooth muscle cells. The majority, however, were stellate and did not stain well with any of the cell-specific antibody markers available. At present, identification of these cells remains uncertain, although it is likely that they are proliferated intimal

Figure 1.20
Potential sources of PDGF in atherogenesis.

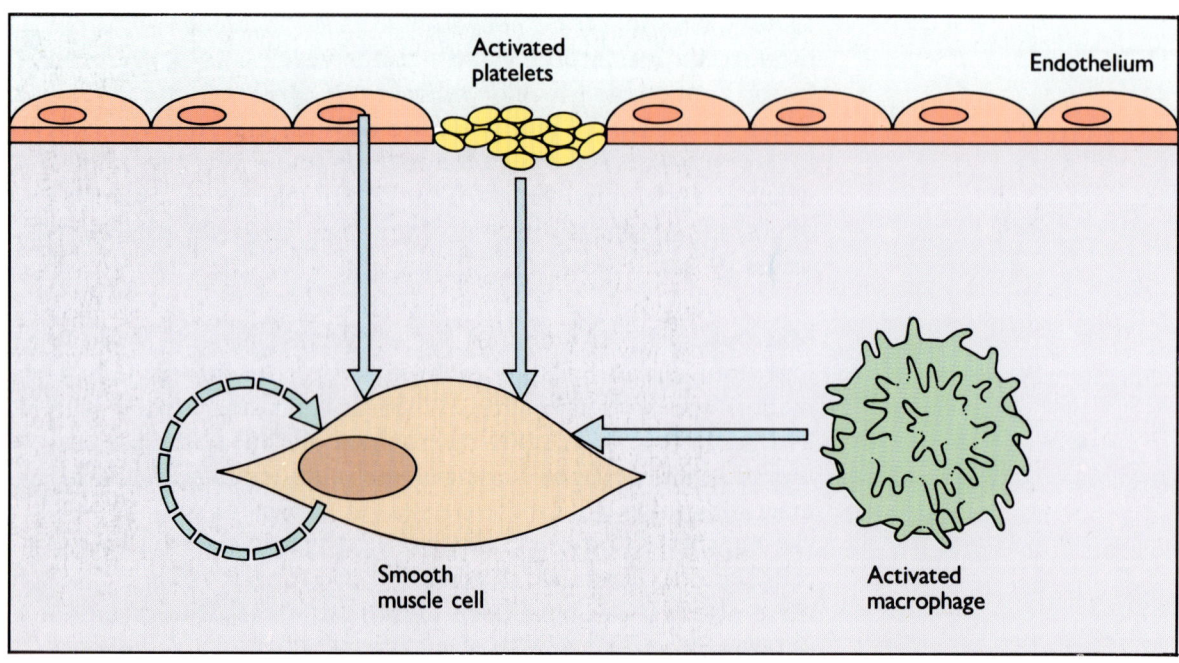

smooth muscle cells. Wilcox and co-workers found no evidence of PDGF mRNA in plaque macrophages, although Barrett and Benditt (103) found that, in atherosclerotic plaques, PDGF B-chain mRNA levels correlated strongly with *fms* mRNA levels (*fms* is the cellular proto-oncogene which codes for the colony stimulating factor-I receptor and is regarded by some as a cell-specific marker for macrophages).

In the Wilcox study, the same arterial samples were hybridized with a PDGF-receptor probe. Many of the cells in the plaques showed mRNA for the receptor; nearly all of these were within the intima and showed the same 'mesenchymal' morphology described above. No cells resembling endothelium or lymphocytes and virtually no foam cells or haemosiderin-containing cells were positive for the PDGF-receptor probe. Those cells which did show mRNA for the PDGF receptor did not react with antibody markers for endothelial cells, lymphocytes or monocytes/macrophages. Few receptor-positive cells were found in the media of the arterial samples examined, a noteworthy observation (see Box).

> According to Wilcox and colleagues, the differential expression of the PDGF receptor within the intima and the media "...establishes the presence of a target in the part of the vessel wall known to undergo selective proliferation in atherosclerosis and following intimal injury such as occurs in the course of angioplasty."

These data, some of which are conflicting, suggest that the chemical regulation of smooth muscle cell migration, proliferation and function in the arterial wall, and the increase in connective tissue resulting from ligand receptor-induced changes in smooth muscle phenotypes, are likely to be very complex phenomena *in vivo* (see Box).

> As summarized by Barrett and Benditt (103): "The findings are consistent with the possibility that the regulation of smooth muscle cell proliferation in atherosclerosis is multifactorial, involving inducers and suppressors, and could centre on a 'cytokine network' of intercellular signalling factors, including immune modulators and peptide growth factors, as well as other substances."

Clonality of smooth muscle cells in atherosclerotic lesions

The data (see above) relating to the interaction between growth factors and intimal smooth muscle cells which results,

it is believed, in the latter expressing their 'synthetic' phenotype suggest that these processes are, in a broad sense, a reaction to injury (74). However, an alternative view has been proposed by Benditt and Benditt (105), who have shown that, in
many instances, the smooth muscle population within mature
atherosclerotic plaques is monotypic and, they believe, monoclonal. They suggest, therefore, that the smooth muscle cell
proliferation in atherogenesis is more closely allied to that in
neoplasia than to that in the repair phase following injury.

This approach to the question of the cell population in
atherosclerotic plaques in man stems from the well known
Lyon hypothesis (106). Mary Lyon, as a result of her studies in
the mouse, showed that, in mammalian females, one of the two
X chromosomes in any diploid cell is largely inactivated and
that the progeny of each cell express the same active X chromosomes as do their parent cells. Since the X-chromosome in-
activation is random, each mammalian female is, in a sense, a
phenotypic mosaic, with individual cells containing either an
active paternal or an active maternal X chromosome. This is
of no consequence in most instances, since the X chromosomes
code for the same proteins. However, the enzyme glucose-6-
phosphate dehydrogenase (G-6-PD) is a special case. This occurs in at least two isoenzymic forms (A and B) which are
easily separated by electrophoresis. In the US, approximately
one-third of Afro-American females are heterozygous for G-
6-PD and individual cells from these women show the presence of either the A or the B isoenzyme, but never both. This
finding is consistent with the Lyon hypothesis. If, therefore, a
lesion characterized by cell proliferation were monoclonal in
origin, only one isoenzyme would be found in the cell population. This was shown to be the case in a study of uterine
leiomyomata derived from Afro-American females heterozygous for G-6-PD (107).

Examination of fibrous aortic plaques from such females for
their isoenzyme composition by the Benditts yielded essentially similar results. In portions of macroscopically normal intima, both the A and B isoenzymes were found. In contrast,
in the vast majority of fibrous plaques examined, only one
isoenzyme was present. From these data, the conclusion was
drawn that this represented a monoclonal expansion of the
smooth muscle cell population; similar observations have been
reported by other groups (108-111).

It is possible that the monotypic nature of the cell population in a plaque may have an explanation other than mono-
clonality. One of the alternative mechanisms considered is the
possibility that the enzyme variant itself or a gene linked by
location on the X chromosome has conferred a selective advantage to the cells; another possibility is that lesion-free clus-
ters of some cells are so large that, if multiplication were trig-
gered, the resulting mass would be monotypic. A further pos-

sibility is that repetitive sampling of the cell population during cycles of cell multiplication and cell death may lead to a drift towards a monotypic population (112). This last suggestion gains some support from the studies of Zavala and associates (113) who cultured fibroblasts from 29 Afro-American females heterozygous for G-6-PD through multiple passages. In 19 of these women, culture revealed only one phenotype. In the remaining 10, the cultures died out while still ditypic.

Hares heterozygous for G-6-PD have been produced by crossing *Lepus europaeus* with *Lepus timidus*. These hybrid hares develop atherosclerotic lesions when maintained on a high cholesterol 'atherogenic' diet (114, 115). The arterial lesions have been examined for their content of the G-6-PD isoenzymes at intervals ranging from three months to two years and, in most, there have been shifts away from the ratio of the isoenzymes found in samples of normal arterial tissue; in only one hare was a completely monotypic lesion found (114).

If the monotypic nature of the cell population in some plaques is indeed a reflection of monoclonal smooth muscle cell proliferation, then it seems not unlikely that the trigger for this proliferation is a mutagen. It is not without interest that, in human plasma, potentially mutagenic hydrocarbons are carried in the lipoprotein fraction (116) and that at least two samples of human aorta have been shown to contain a mixed-function oxidase system (aryl-4-mono-oxygenase) which may transform premutagens into substances that are cytotoxic, or may attach themselves to substances covalently to DNA and bring about modification (117).

There is experimental evidence to support such a genesis of some plaques. Herpesvirus mRNA has been shown to be present by hybridization in cells of human atherosclerotic plaques (118). Weekly injections of carcinogenic hydrocarbons have resulted in the appearance of fibromuscular plaques in the abdominal aortas of cockerels (119); 15-week-old cockerels, injected at the age of four days with the oncogenic Marek's disease virus, developed focal microscopic plaques in the thoracic aorta (120, 121).

An experiment of great potential significance in relation to the monoclonal hypothesis has been the demonstration by Penn and colleagues (119), who found that DNA extracted from samples of some human coronary artery plaques contained a transforming gene. The assay used relies on the incorporation and expression of dominant transforming DNA sequences by NIH 3T3 cells, an immortalized murine fibroblast line which has proved susceptible to transformation by genes of the *ras* group. The morphological correlate of such transformation is the appearance in monolayer cultures of foci of 3T3 cells wherein the cells are heaped together (presumably having lost contact inhibition) and the individual cells are smaller and rounder than those of the surrounding monolayer. DNA from such foci must be able to produce the same changes in other 3T3 cultures; the final proof that transformation has occurred is provided by assessing the ability of cells from the 'foci' to produce tumours when injected into suitable hosts, most notably the athymic 'nude' mouse (Figure 1.21). Samples from three groups of human coronary artery plaque DNA gave rise to transformed foci when transfected into 3T3 cells, while DNA samples from a variety of non-malignant tissues, including coronary artery, failed to do so. Southern-blotted DNA from the transformed foci yielded positive signals when hybridized to a ^{32}P-labelled, nick-translated, repetitive human *alu* sequence, indicating the presence of human genetic material, but no active *ras* oncogenes were seen. Primary focus cells from each of five clones produced slowly growing tu-

Figure 1.21
Results of an in-vitro and in-vivo study indicate that some plaques in man contain transformine factors (Penn et al, 1986).

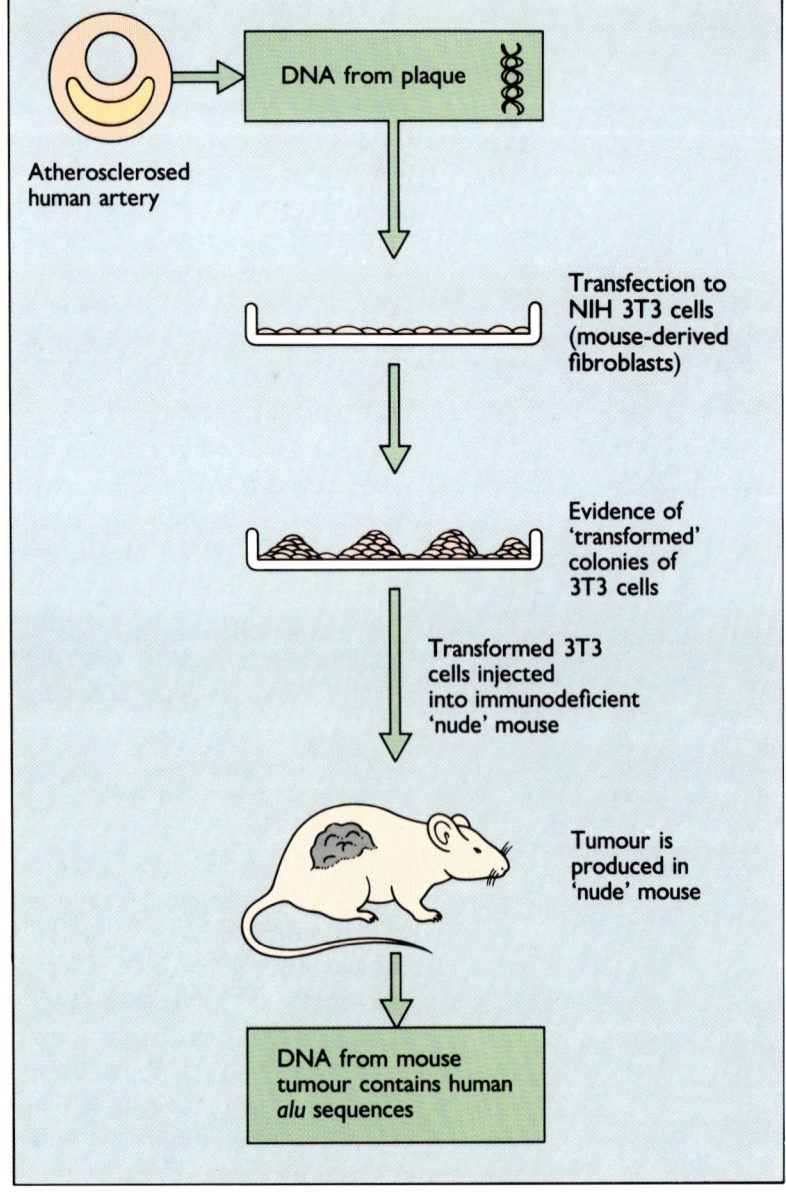

mours in 6/42 nude mice, and samples of the tumour DNA also hybridized to *alu*. These data suggest that somatic gene alterations can play a significant role in the genesis of some atherosclerotic plaques.

Intimal lipid accumulation

As in most mammalian tissues, the artery wall contains a considerable amount of lipid which increases with normal growth and ageing (122,123). Such increases on ageing are brought about, in part, by a slow and steady increase in free cholesterol, triglyceride and phospholipid concentrations. The concentration of esterified cholesterol within the vessel wall remains low well into the second decade of life, then rises very rapidly so that, in normal arterial intima from patients aged 40 to 59 years, cholesteryl ester makes up more than 40% of the total lipid content.

Atherosclerotic lesions contain far more lipid than does normal arterial intima; for example, fatty streaks contain approximately nine times as much lipid as the lesion-free aorta in children and adolescents and nearly four times as much as in subjects aged between 40 to 59 years. Between 65 to 80% of this lipid is cholesterol, and the ratio of esterified to free cholesterol is high in most lesions (124). The cholesterol fatty acid pattern in juvenile fatty streaks differs from that in both plasma and fibrolipid plaques, where the principal fatty acid is linoleic acid. Cholesteryl ester in juvenile fatty streaks contains large amounts of oleate and relatively little linoleate (125-127). The greater the number of foam cells in the fatty streaks, the greater the difference appears to be. This suggests that the cholesteryl ester of the fatty streak is derived from esterification of the cholesterol within the foam cells.

The cholesteryl esters accumulating within the arterial intima are believed to originate from the circulating lipoproteins which enter the interstitial spaces of the artery wall (128). En-

Figure 1.22
Histology of the cap of an aortic plaque treated with a fluorescein-linked polyclonal antibody to LDL. The presence of apoprotein is indicated by the numerous areas of fluorescence within the thickened intima.

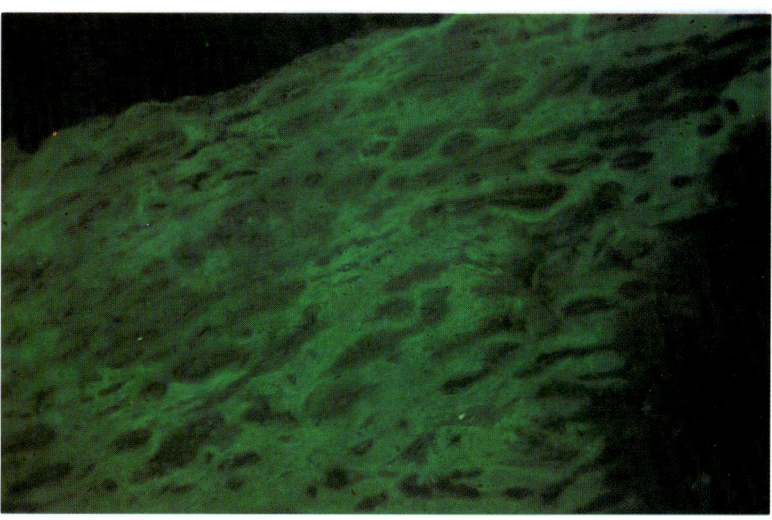

try can be effected either by the formation of an ultrafiltrate of plasma or by transcytosis of LDL through the endothelial cells.

That the origin of plaque cholesterol is from plasma lipoprotein is supported by the immunohistochemical demonstration of apoproteins within atherosclerotic lesions (55,129-132) (Figure 1.22). Smith and Slater (133) developed an elegant microimmunoassay method for quantifying lipoprotein within the vessel wall, consisting of electrophoresis of lipoprotein directly from minced portions of artery wall into a gel containing antilipoprotein globulin. The resulting antigen-antibody complex precipitates as a rocket-shaped peak and the area beneath it is proportional to the amount of extractable antigen. Using this method, a high degree of correlation was found between the amount of lipoprotein extractable from the artery wall and the plasma cholesterol concentration of the same patient in the week preceding death (123).

The fate of the lipoprotein entering the arterial intima is now much better understood, mostly due to the discovery of the LDL-receptor pathway by Brown and Goldstein (134-137) (Figure 1.23) and to the recognition that the majority of foam cells in fatty streaks are macrophages.

More than 60% of LDL clearance from the plasma is mediated through binding to the LDL receptor and subsequent endocytosis (see 'Hyperlipidaemia as a risk factor for atheroscle-

Figure 1.23
LDL enters the subendothelial space and undergoes oxidative modification through lipoxygenase-mediated metabolism, resulting in both the lipid and apoprotein moieties of arachidonic acid. Modified from Brown and Goldstein, 1988, with permission.

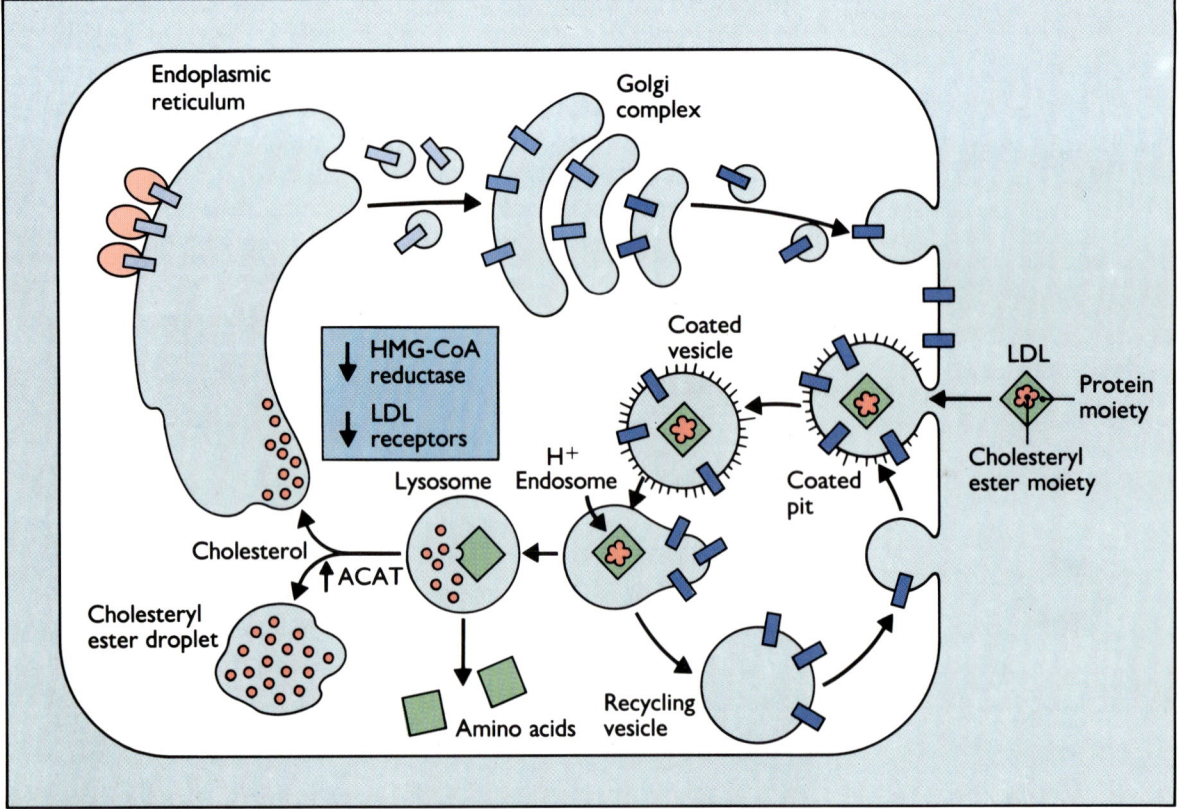

rosis'), most of which takes place as a result of ligand-receptor binding within the liver. In the artery wall, however, available evidence suggests that the LDL receptor is not a major factor in the handling of the LDL which reaches the intima (138). The Watanabe heritable hyperlipidaemic (WHHL) rabbit develops fatty streaks rich in foam cells, even though it is totally devoid of LDL receptors (14,139). In addition, normal monocytes and monocyte-derived macrophages in culture are not converted into foam cells by incubation with unmodified LDL (140,141). However, chemically modified LDL is avidly taken up by monocytes in cell culture. This is believed to be due to another receptor called the 'scavenger receptor'. This receptor does not recognize unmodified LDL, but binds LDL which has been either acetylated or conjugated with malondialdehyde, an aldehyde product of lipid peroxidation (142).

Oxidative modification of LDL

If LDL is incubated in the presence of cultured endothelial cells, arterial smooth muscle cells or macrophages, it undergoes extensive modification (143-145), the most striking of which is the ability to bind to the scavenger receptor on macrophages and, thus, to undergo endocytosis and intracellular degradation. On modification, the LDL is no longer recognized by the LDL receptor. In addition, the modified LDL becomes a strong chemoattractant for human monocytes (in man) because of alterations in the lipid moiety of the LDL, in particular, the accumulation of significant amounts of lysolecithin (146-148). Not only does the altered LDL act as a chemotactic signal for monocytes but, in mice, it also inhibits the basal motility of peritoneal macrophages and their ability to respond to other chemotactic agents. As many studies of the effects of hyperlipidaemia on the artery wall suggest that one of the earliest events morphologically is the adhesion of white cells to the endothelial surface, followed by entry into the subjacent intima, this chemotactic effect of modified LDL may be a primary event in the genesis of the fatty streak (138,149).

Nature of LDL modification

The changes that occur in the LDL molecule, whether following incubation with one of the cell types mentioned above or incubation with plasma containing copper or iron, depend on peroxidation of polyunsaturated fatty acids in the lipid fraction and, thus, on free-radical generation either by endothelial cells or monocyte/macrophages. This is shown by the fact that LDL modification by endothelial cells is blocked if the incubation takes place in the presence of antioxidants, such as vitamin E or butylated hydroxytoluene. Modification of LDL involves changes in both the lipid and protein moieties (Figure 1.24). In the lipid moiety, there is a significant degree of conversion of lecithin to lysolecithin, and the cytotoxic effects of modified

LDL on endothelial cells in culture is probably largely dependent on this (150,151). However, in the course of peroxidation of unsaturated lipid moieties, 4-hydroxyalkenals can be generated from omega-6- and omega-3-polyunsaturated fatty acids; these compounds, which are very active biologically, can cause severe disturbances of cell function at a number of levels (152). Steinbrecher (154) has shown that cleavage products of arachidonic acid may react with apoprotein B, a reaction which involves blocking of the epsilon-amino groups of lysine residues. It is now believed that the interaction of aldehydic lipid peroxidation products with these epsilon-amino groups of lysine residues produces new epitopes which are recognized by the scavenger receptors on macrophages (153). Thus, the generation of free radicals in the subendothelial space may have a variety of important results (see Box):

Cytotoxic chemical species may form which play a role in the later stages of plaque evolution;

Foam cell formation may be mediated through the scavenger receptor;

Monocytes may be attracted to the intima involved and become immobilized.

Does oxidation of LDL occur in vivo?
However interesting the ex-vivo data (see above), it is important to ascertain whether these reactions occur in 'real life'. There are two conceptual starting points (see Box).

If oxidative modification of LDL plays a role in atherogenesis, does the use of appropriate antioxidants at appropriate dosages inhibit the genesis and progression of atherosclerotic lesions?

This proposition has been demonstrated (155,156) in an animal model with probucol, an antioxidant which has a mildly hypolipidaemic action, administered to hypercholesterolaemic WHHL rabbits. There was marked inhibition of lesion development and apparently with little effect on plasma lipid concentrations.

Does examination of the arterial lesions themselves reveal evidence of oxidative modification of LDL?

Haberland, Fong and Cheng (157) were the first to show that antibodies prepared against malondialdehyde-modified LDL bound to antigens present within the lipid-rich lesions in the aortas of WHHL rabbits and that this antigen co-localized with apoB-100 protein in these lesions. These results have been confirmed by Palinski and associates (158), who also found that LDL extracted from lesions in the WHHL rabbits is recognized by an antiserum prepared against malondialdehyde-conjugated LDL, and that autoantibodies against malondialdehyde-modified LDL can be found in both rabbit and human sera.

Other roles for the macrophage in atherosclerotic lesions

Earlier in this chapter, the possibility was discussed that the macrophage, as a result of its ability to synthesize PDGF, may play a role in stimulating smooth muscle cell proliferation in atherogenesis. Similarly, there is apparently a nexus between LDL oxidation in the subendothelial space, chemo-attraction of monocytes and the formation of foam cells following lipid uptake by the so-called scavenger receptors (Figure 1.24). The activated macrophage synthesizes and secretes a wide range of active cytokines, thus acquiring a dominant role in modulating events in the course of inflammation and healing. It is not unreasonable, then, to examine the possibility that the macrophage may play a similar role in the evolution of atherosclerotic plaques.

The macrophage may, for example, produce both inter-leukin-1 (IL-1) and tumour necrosis factor (TNF). Both of these cytokines have a wide range of biological effects but, in the context of atherogenesis, the effect of these two compounds on vascular endothelium is of particular interest. Both TNF and IL-1 cause the expression of adhesion molecules on the endothelial cell surface which are capable of producing leucocyte/endothelial cell adhesion (159-161). In addition, the macrophage secretes a large number of chemotactic factors (162). The combination of these two functions may act as a recruitment mechanism for the macrophage population within a plaque.

IL-1 may also act as a mitogenic factor while TNF is angio-genic, which may account for the transmedial ingrowth of new capillaries seen in large plaques.

Also of interest is the possibility that the macrophage may contribute to basal necrosis, a key element in the natural history of many lesions in man. Tissue damage may occur both within the plaque substance and at the endothelial surface as a result of the release by activated macrophages of oxygen-free radicals; it is noteworthy that such free-radical release is

Figure 1.24
LDL receptor pathway: LDL receptors bind LDL and deliver it to lysosomes for degradation. After endocytosis, the receptors return to the cell surface to bind another LDL. Modified from Brown and Goldstein, 1985, with permission.

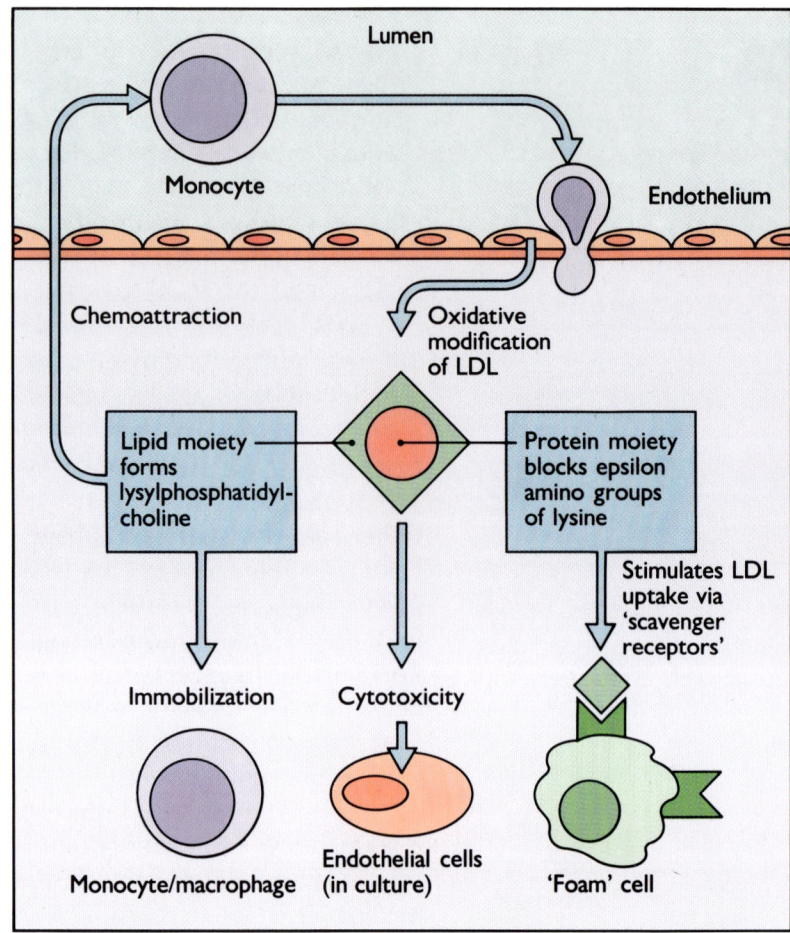

potentiated (ex-vivo) by exposure of macrophages to oxidized LDL (163). Macrophages may also release powerful proteases, including collagenase and elastase, either by reverse endocytosis or as a result of macrophage death; this, too, may play a part in the connective tissue necrosis believed to occur at the plaque base. However, these observations are primarily derived from cell culture studies and, thus, should be treated with caution, although further studies of the role of the multifunctional macrophage both in plaque genesis and in the later natural history of the lesion are appropriate.

T lymphocytes within plaques: Possible interactions
As already described, adventitial collections of lymphocytes are common and probably represent a reaction to antigenic components derived from the lipid-rich atheromatous pool. However, recent immunohistochemical studies of plaque cell populations have shown that, in addition to smooth muscle cells and macrophages, T lymphocytes are also present (164).

In a study involving plaques removed from the human internal carotid artery during surgery, a panel of monoclonal antibodies was used to identify the different cell types present.

Macrophages, as identified by the antibody anti-leu-M3,

were found throughout the plaque, but were concentrated within the lipid-rich basal pool, constituting 60% of the cell population. Cells expressing the CD3 antigen, which identifies T cells, were most abundant in the fibrous cap, constituting 20% of the cells present. The correctness of this identification was established by isolating cells from the plaques by collagenase digestion and performing a variety of functional assays. Some of these cells (approximately 5%) showed the rosetting activity typical of T cells.

In other studies, the same workers found that smooth muscle cells of atherosclerotic lesions express class II MHC antigens (HLA-DR and HLA-DQ), which are absent from normal arterial intima (165,166). These antigens are inducible on smooth muscle cells in culture by the T-cell product gamma interferon, and their presence may be interpreted as evidence that interactions between the immune system and elements of the vessel wall are involved in atherogenesis (167). Similar findings have been reported by Emeson and Robertson (168), who showed that both T-helper (CD4) and T-suppressor (CD8) cells can be identified within plaques; they have suggested that activated T cells may be instrumental in amplifying the mechanisms responsible for attracting monocytes to sites where atherogenesis is in progress.

Factors affecting the extent and severity of atherosclerosis

The major differences in the prevalence of atherosclerosis-related clinical disease between countries provide an opportunity for international comparisons of the causal factors suspected in these diseases (169). It is to be expected that some factors will be found to be more consistently associated with clinical expressions of atherosclerosis than others; these may be further studied both for the strength of their association and for modifications which may relate to changes in population trends for such diseases.

Within a given population in which atherosclerosis-related disease is endemic, for example in the UK, there may be considerable regional differences. Scotland and the North of England have death rates from ischaemic heart disease which are twice as high as those in the South East of England. Within Scotland, rates are much higher in the western than eastern regions, with a two-fold difference between the highest and lowest rates; within a single city (for example, Glasgow), there are areas in which the death rate from ischaemic heart disease is twice as high as in others (169). Major clinical events, for example, myocardial infarction, are the result of a number of interdependent factors of which the extent and severity of atherosclerosis is only one. However, in the vast majority of cases, arterial occlusion or a significant degree of arterial narowing does not occur in the absence of atherosclerosis.

Atherosclerosis is **necessary**, if not always **sufficient**, to bring about a major occlusive event. It is both reasonable and correct to assess the effects on extent and severity of atherosclerosis of recognized high-risk factors for major artery-related syndromes.

Relationship between atherosclerosis and occlusive arterial disease

To determine the value of assessing the effect of individual risk factors for CHD on, for example, atherosclerosis, it is necessary to establish the degree of correlation between the extent and severity of atherosclerosis and the prevalence of CHD in a given population. This is 'easier said than done' as there are serious methodological and conceptual difficulties in quantifying atherosclerosis (170,171) (see Box).

How best to measure the extent and severity of atherosclerosis? More important, how to define more or less severe atherosclerosis? Does this refer to a greater or lesser area of involvement of the arterial intima, or does this relate to the prevalence and extent of a more specific morphological variation, such as a soft, lipid-rich eccentric plaque at a specific location within the arterial system?

As regards the methods used in various attempts to quantify atherosclerosis, the subject has been reviewed by Woolf (171) and included in the International Atherosclerosis Project (IAP), published in 1968 as a supplement to *Laboratory Investigation*. The IAP was a collaborative study carried out in the 1960s with the objective to grade atherosclerosis in five different arterial beds in populations drawn from 19 different locations. The racial groups studied included whites, blacks, Asian Indians, American Indians and mulattos. Some of these groups had a high prevalence of CHD while, in others, it was low. Altogether, 23,000 sets of vessels were studied, leading to the significant result that (see Box):

There is a strong predictive value of the mature fibrolipid plaque or raised lesion for death due to CHD (38,39).

Consistent with this, the decline in mortality due to CHD in the US (172) has been accompanied, according to the necropsy survey carried out by Strong and Guzman (173), by a significant reduction in the frequency and size of fibrolipid plaques in the coronary arteries.

Risk factors and atherosclerosis

What is a risk factor? Stamler and his colleagues (174) have defined it as a "... habit, trait or abnormality associated with a sizeable increase in susceptibility to disease associated with severe or extensive atherosclerosis." The risk-factor concept is important as significant progress in controlling atherosclerosis-related disease is likely to be made only if severe atherosclerosis is prevented – so-called primary prevention; this can only be achieved by the identification of risk factors which are either avoidable or reversible. However, it may be that some of the factors found to be epidemiologically related to the prevalence of arterial disease may not have a direct causal relationship and, thus, removal or reversal of such a factor will have no effect. Furthermore, not all factors epidemiologically related to the prevalence of arterial disease can be described as a "habit, trait or abnormality" unless age, gender and race can be so regarded. In any consideration of the natural history of atherosclerosis, these latter variables require careful examination.

Age

Of all factors considered to affect atherogenesis, age has the strongest and most consistent association. Lesions appear in the aorta in the first decade of life, in the coronary arteries in the second and in the cerebral arteries in the third (175).

Robertson's data indicate that the aorta is the site of the most rapid development of mature lesions while the cerebral arteries are the site of the least rapid development, and the coronary arteries are in an intermediate position. Fatty streaks occupy approximately 10% of the aortic intimal surface by the age of 10 years and may increase, reaching a peak of 28 to 30% by the age of 30 years. After this point, the extent of involvement by fatty streaks does not increase and, indeed, often decreases. This may be due in part to the 'replacement' of some fatty streaks by raised lesions and in part to regression of lesions. In contrast, fibrolipid plaques first appear in the aorta in the third decade of life and increase progressively with age. It is not possible to say whether ageing itself is implicated in atherogenesis or whether the effects of age represent a longer period of action by other factors, such as hyperlipidaemia, hypertension, diabetes or cigarette-smoking.

Gender

Large-scale epidemiological studies have indicated that CHD during the middle decades of life is far less common in women than in men. With increasing age, this gender difference gradually decreases, but never completely disappears. These data are, in part, reflected by studies of the prevalence and severity of atherosclerosis in the two sexes. In the IAP study, male gender was associated with a greater extent of coronary involvement by advanced fibrolipid plaques, although this was not seen in the aorta. The gender difference in the coronary arteries was much greater in white than in black subjects (37,176). Removing all cases with other identifiable risk factors from the IAP series, insofar as is possible *post mortem*, did not eliminate the gender difference in coronary plaques. McGill (177) suggested that this finding corresponds with epidemiological data showing that risk factors are less predictive for CHD in women than in men.

It is tempting to speculate that female hormones are responsible for the epidemiological differences in atherogenesis and CHD which appear to operate in favour of women during their reproductive phase. Numerous experiments have been carried out in a variety of animal species to assess whether oestrogens have an effect on the induction of atherosclerosis by dietary and/or pharmacological means. Many of the data obtained are contradictory and, as they have been derived primarily in small animal species not known for their propensity to develop atherosclerosis spontaneously, it is difficult to know what significance to attach to them.

In man, the use of oestrogens in a secondary prevention trial has not been encouraging. Myocardial infarction was significantly more frequent in the 'treatment' group than in those receiving placebo, as were thrombophlebitis and non-fatal pulmonary embolism (178). However, this does not negate the fact that female gender is protective, although further studies are needed to analyze the mechanisms responsible.

There appear to be differences between the sexes in lipid metabolism. Post-heparin lipoprotein lipase activity is greater in women than in men (179), and mean concentrations of high-density lipoprotein (HDL) cholesterol have been found to be higher in women (57.94 mg/dl) than in men (42.40 mg/dl) (180).

Race

As already stated, there are striking geographical differences in the prevalence of CHD and these are mirrored by similar differences in the extent of intimal involvement by fibrolipid plaques. In the IAP study there was, for instance (with the single exception of females in New Orleans), less atherosclerosis in the form of fibrolipid plaques in the negro populations studied than in whites. In three locations in which both white and negro populations were studied the negro moiety of the necropsy population showed much less atherosclerosis than the white and, in Durban, where members of three racial groups formed the sample, negroes showed less atherosclerosis than either whites or Asian Indians. The moot point is whether these observed differences are mediated by racial differences or environmental (which one can interpret as socioeconomic) factors. Within each racial group studied, there is a strong gradient for coronary atherosclerosis and this suggests that belonging to a particular racial group does not in itself confer either relative immunity from or increased susceptibility to atherosclerosis. This view is strengthened by data gained from studies of immigrant populations. Keys (181) compared the prevalence of CHD among Japanese resident in Japan and those resident either in Hawaii or in the USA. The expatriates showed a far higher frequency of CHD than their compatriots in Japan. In this connexion, it is interesting to compare the distribution of plasma cholesterol concentrations in Japanese men living in Japan and those living in California. It is true to say that there was a higher prevalence of hypercholesterolaemia in those living in California, but this statement gives an incomplete picture of the state of affairs – the whole distribution curve for those living in California was shifted to the right as compared with those living in Japan (182).

Hyperlipidaemia and atherosclerosis

There is a vast literature which relates to the association between lipid metabolism, atherosclerosis and clinically significant arterial disease. Despite the complexity of this subject, this association may be expressed in a series of simple propositions, each of which requires careful and critical examination (see Box).

Atherosclerotic lesions contain far more lipid of certain subclasses than adjacent areas of normal intima.

The production of raised plasma concentrations of certain lipids in a variety of experimental animals by dietary and/or pharmacological means is followed by the appearance of arterial lesions which have some features in common with human atherosclerosis. Strains of rabbits with hyperlipidaemia occurring on a genetic basis also develop arterial lesions.

An association exists between populations in whom the prevalence of CHD and of fibrolipid plaques is high and high plasma concentrations of certain lipids, most notably LDL cholesterol in populations in which CHD is prevalent. For example, in two villages where mean total plasma cholesterol was approximately 4 mmol/l, the incidence of CHD was reported as being less than 5/1000 men/10 years. In eastern Finland, where the mean total cholesterol concentration was just under 7 mmol/l, the incidence of fatal coronary events was 14 times as high. The converse applies when the prevalence of CHD and fibrolipid plaques is low. This association is especially strong in patients with particular genetically determined hyperlipidaemias, such as familial hypercholesterolaemia, in which a single gene defect leads to a large increase in cholesterol-rich atherogenic LDL, premature atherosclerosis and coronary heart disease.

Prospective epidemiological studies have established that the higher the plasma concentrations of LDL cholesterol, the greater the risk of CHD. Similarly, there are data now available from a number of studies indicating that lowering LDL-cholesterol concentrations reduces the risk of a major coronary event.

Plasma lipid concentrations and atherosclerosis
The extent of intimal involvement by atherosclerosis appears to be related both to total plasma cholesterol and dietary fat intake when different populations are compared, although Strong, Eggen and Oalmann (176) maintained that there were no data showing a positive association between atherosclerosis, diet and plasma lipids within a single population. Shekelle and colleagues (183), however, in their long-running Western Electric study, have demonstrated that there is a positive association between dietary fat intake and plasma cholesterol concentration within a relatively homogeneous population sample. The Oslo study (184), based on necropsy material, showed that while there is wide individual variation in involvement by fibrolipid plaques, both the mean and median values for such lesions increase with increasing plasma total cholesterol concentrations during life; similar data are reported from other necropsy-based studies in single populations.

Genetically determined hyperlipidaemias
'Experiments of nature' in the form of genetically determined hyperlipoproteinaemia have helped to confirm the association between hyperlipidaemia and CHD (185).

Familial hypercholesterolaemia (FH). This is the result of a quantitative or qualitative abnormality in a receptor for apoproteins B and E that is normally found on the surface of many cells, most notably liver cells, as described in 1973 by the

Nobel laureates Michael Brown and Joseph Goldstein (186). The receptor, coded for by a gene on chromosome 19, is a single-protein chain which spans the plasma membrane (Figure 1.25). The outer portion contains the binding site for LDL, and the inner portion which projects into the cytoplasm contains the signal mechanisms that enable the bound LDL to be carried into the cell by receptor-mediated endocytosis (187). The receptors are clustered within discrete indentations in the plasma membrane coated by a protein called clathrin. These 'coated pits' are the gateway for the entry of LDL molecules into the cell. Such concentration of the receptors is a function of their intracytoplasmic portions without which LDL cannot be endocytosed even though it may bind to the outer portion of the receptor. LDL transport into the cell is mediated by invagination of the coated pit which is then 'pinched off' from the plasma membrane to form a membrane-bound vesicle. Fusion takes place between the LDL-containing vesicle and a lysosome, and the receptor splits from the LDL to be recycled to the surface where it can bind with another LDL particle. Each receptor migrates into and out of the cytoplasm once every 10 minutes (see Figure 1.23).

In most populations, approximately 1/500 have one mutant gene for the LDL receptor. These subjects are heterozygous

Figure 1.25
Diagrammatic representation of the structure of the LDL receptor, established through cloning and sequencing of a complementary DNA. Of the five domains, the most important is 1, which binds LDL, and 5, which directs the receptor to coated pits. From Brown and Goldstein, 1986, with permission.

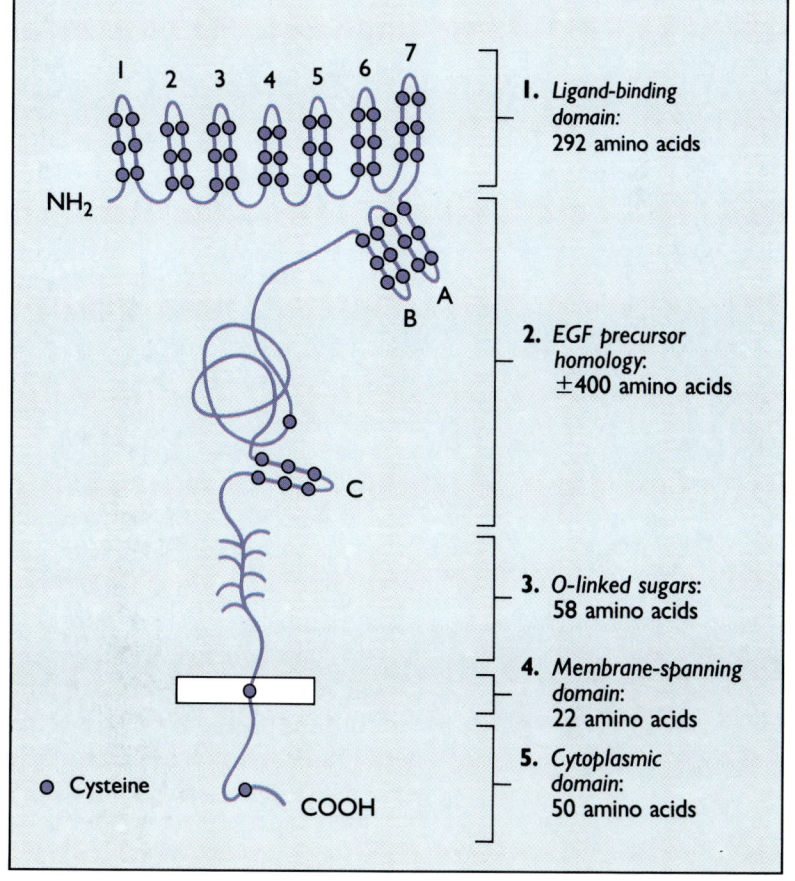

1. *Ligand-binding domain:* 292 amino acids

2. *EGF precursor homology:* ±400 amino acids

3. *O-linked sugars:* 58 amino acids

4. *Membrane-spanning domain:* 22 amino acids

5. *Cytoplasmic domain:* 50 amino acids

○ Cysteine

for familial hypercholesterolaemia and produce only half the normal number of LDL receptors. Their plasma LDL concentrations are elevated (approximately twice normal levels), and they have an increased risk of developing major coronary events in their fourth and fifth decades.

Fortunately very rare (1/1,000,000) are homozygotes who inherit two copies of mutant LDL-receptor genes. The likelihood of two heterozygotes marrying each other is 1/250,000; their children have an approximately six-fold greater LDL-cholesterol concentration and develop severe atherosclerosis very early in life and typically suffer from CHD before the age of 20 years or earlier.

> *"Homozygous FH is a vivid experiment of nature. It demonstrates unequivocally the causal relation between an elevated circulating-LDL level and atherosclerosis."*
>
> *Brown and Goldstein (136)*

While homozygous FH is very rare, diet-related hypercholesterolaemia is not. In this condition, LDL-receptor number and function may be vitally important as high-fat diets may lead to a 10 to 20% suppression of LDL receptors, especially on liver cells where excess lipid activates an oxysterol-binding protein which 'switches off' the LDL-receptor gene. Not all subjects receiving a high-fat diet are affected; Brown has suggested that there may be two regulatory responses to dietary fat. In one, the high-fat diet leads to a decrease in cholesterol synthesis, as seen in Pima Indians, who have a very high-fat diet, but are not hypercholesterolaemic. In the other, the high-fat diet leads to a partial suppression of LDL receptors and, thus, to hypercholesterolaemia.

Familial combined hyperlipidaemia (FCHL). This autosomal dominant disorder is characterized by a variety of abnormal plasma lipoprotein patterns within affected families. Patients may have isolated hypercholesterolaemia, a combination of hypercholesterolaemia and hypertriglyceridaemia or, in about one-third of cases, hypertriglyceridaemia alone. Affected individuals have an increased risk of CHD. In one study, FCHL was found to be the most common genetic dyslipidaemia in first-degree relatives of patients aged less than 50 years who had had a myocardial infarct; in addition, approximately 15% of patients experiencing a major coronary event before reaching the age of 60 years apparently have this disorder.

The metabolic defect appears to be an overproduction of apoprotein B-100 by the liver, and the resulting very low-density lipoprotein (VLDL) particles are small, rich in apoB-100 and possibly atherogenic (185).

Familial dysbetalipoproteinaemia. This relatively uncommon condition has a frequency rate of about 1/5000 persons in the US. Also known as Type 3 hyperlipoproteinaemia, it involves delayed catabolism of VLDL remnants and chylomicrons, and the plasma contains an abnormal form of VLDL (beta-VLDL) which is abnormally rich in cholesterol. These individuals are homozygous for an isomorphic form of apolipoprotein E ($apoE_2$) which binds less avidly to its receptor than the more common $apoE_3$. For hyperlipidaemia to develop in these subjects, an additional metabolic defect must be present, as approximately 15% of the population are homozygous for $apoE_2$, yet most are not hyperlipidaemic. If hyperlipidaemia is present, there is an increased risk both of premature CHD and peripheral vascular disease. Such subjects are frequently obese, glucose intolerant, hyperuricaemic, and have tuboeruptive and palmar xanthomas. Their triglyceride concentrations are often somewhat higher than those of cholesterol (although both are markedly increased), with the latter in the VLDL fraction.

Plasma triglycerides and cardiovascular disease
The relationship between plasma triglyceride concentrations and cardiovascular disease is controversial. Although hypertriglyceridaemia is positively associated with risk in most population studies, with adjustment for total- and HDL-cholesterol concentrations, cigarette-smoking and high blood pressure, for example, the association becomes weaker. In the Framingham study, however, the plasma triglyceride concentration was found to be an independent predictor of CHD in women. Indeed, diseases associated with elevated plasma triglyceride concentrations, such as diabetes mellitus, nephrotic syndrome and chronic renal disorders, increased the risk of CHD (188).

Effects of hyperlipidaemia on artery wall
Since the initial experiments by Anitschkow and Chalatow in 1913 (189) in which they induced intimal lesions in the aorta of rabbits by means of a diet rich in egg yolk, numerous studies have been performed to investigate the effects of increasing the concentrations of specific lipids in the blood of different animal species through dietary and/or pharmacological means. More recently, the introduction of SEM, which permits the examination of large areas of vascular surfaces at a wide range of magnifications, has not only decreased the sampling errors inherent in other histopathological techniques, but allowed identification of the changes in the vessel wall which antedate the development of atherosclerotic lesions.

Effects of diet-induced hyperlipidaemia in primates
Of the many studies of the effects of diet-induced hyperlipidaemia on the artery wall, that of Faggiotto and colleagues

(13,27) carried out in primates profited from SEM examination. Hypercholesterolaemia was induced in primates (*Macaca nemestrina*) by a diet containing 42% fat supplemented with 0.5 g of cholesterol for every 100 g of diet; plasma cholesterol concentrations were between 500 and 1000 mg/dl.

Within 12 days of induction of hyperlipidemia, monocytes could be seen adhering to the intimal surface of the aorta. During the third month, defects appeared in the aortic endothelium, resulting in exposure of the underlying foam cells to circulating blood. The presence of foam cells in smears made from whole blood from these animals suggests that emigration of the lipid-laden macrophages does indeed occur. After four months of hypercholesterolaemia, endothelial defects in the iliac arteries of some of the monkeys were observed to be associated with extensive platelet adherence and the formation of microthrombi. In animals which remained on the high-fat diet for up to thirteen months, well established fibrous plaques with necrotic bases were found. These were most commonly in the abdominal aorta and iliac arteries, particularly in areas of endothelial denudation associated with microthrombus formation. This was the first experimental study in which the events that mediate progression from fatty streaks to fibrous plaques was outlined in detail; it is thus of great significance.

Arterial changes in genetically hyperlipidaemic animals
The discovery of animal strains with inherited abnormalities of lipid metabolism allowed the study of the morphological events of plaque genesis without the use of grossly unphysiological diets. Koletsky (190) isolated an obese mutant from a colony of spontaneously hypertensive rats (SHRs); when homozygous for the cp (corpulent) gene, the animals were both obese and hypertensive, and developed atherosclerosis while receiving a normal diet. A recent study (191) has described the arterial changes in the arteries of a strain derived from the Koletsky rat, the LA/N-corpulent rat, which is both obese and hyperlipidaemic. Numerous lesions were found in the arteries on SEM examination, including desquamation of endothelial cells associated with adherence of platelets and fibrin.

The WHHL rabbit was the first homologue of one of the genetically determined hyperlipidaemias in man to be discovered. This strain exhibits the same deficiency of LDL receptors as in Type IIa hyperlipidaemia (familial hypercholesterolaemia) (192-194). The cellular pathology of the progressive atherosclerosis in this animal model has been described in considerable detail (14,138). The earliest morphologically detectable events in lesion initiation were monocyte adhesion to arterial endothelium, followed by ingress of the monocytes between adjacent endothelial cells and their conversion to foam cells. Further development of these lesions is marked by hypertrophy of the immediately subendothelial foam cells associated with their exposure to the blood as a result, presumably, of endothelial cell retraction. These appearances are identical with those observed in fat-fed rabbits with comparable plasma cholesterol concentrations.

Recently, a strain of New Zealand White (NZW) rabbit (St Thomas' Hospital strain) has been identified in which the pronounced genetically determined hyperlipidaemia is characterized by overproduction of VLDL and LDL (15,195). In this animal model, the LDL-receptor deficiency described in patients with familial hypercholesterolaemia and in the WHHL rabbit is not present, and receptor-mediated catabolism of LDL is normal. Plasma cholesterol concentrations in these animals are markedly elevated; in rabbits more than four months old, cholesterol concentration was 394 ±100 mg/dl (mean ±SD). Cholesterol levels increase during the first three months of life, after which the trend is apparently not age-related. The mean cholesterol concentration in normal male and female NZW rabbits is 77 ±25 mg/dl and 89 ±21 mg/dl respectively. Mean triglyceride concentrations are less markedly raised in the affected animals (151 ±59 mg/dl) than in normal NZW rabbits (84 ±31 mg/dl).

This disorder appears to be transmitted vertically and a range of lipid abnormalities is encountered as a result of matings between hypercholesterolaemic animals. The most common of these is hypercholesterolaemia with normal triglyceride levels, although elevations of triglyceride alone or of both lipid classes also occur. In summary, this strain appears to mimic the features of FCHL.

Arterial pathology in the St Thomas' Hospital strain

On macroscopic examination of the aorta, no lesions can be identified until the affected animals are between four and six months old, after which areas in which much lipid has accumulated are easily identifiable. The region which is earliest and most severely affected is the descending portion of the thoracic aorta, although lesions are present throughout all portions of the aorta. By staining the whole specimen with a mixture of Sudan III and IV, it is relatively easy to map out and measure the extent of intimal surface involvement. In the aortas of severely affected animals, this may be more than 80%. In animals of the same age, the intimal surface area involved correlates well with plasma total cholesterol concentration and with the LDL-cholesterol levels (Figure 1.26).

Light microscopic appearances

Histological examination of the arterial lesions shows a marked increase in intimal thickness involving, in some instances, more than half the circumference of the aorta. In the most severely affected areas, the increase in intimal thickness as compared to that seen in normocholesterolaemic animals of the same

Figure 1.26
Post-mortem section of aorta from an 18-month-old hyperlipidaemic rabbit (St Thomas' Hospital strain). After treatment with a fat-soluble dye, the very extensive lipid deposition appears bright red.

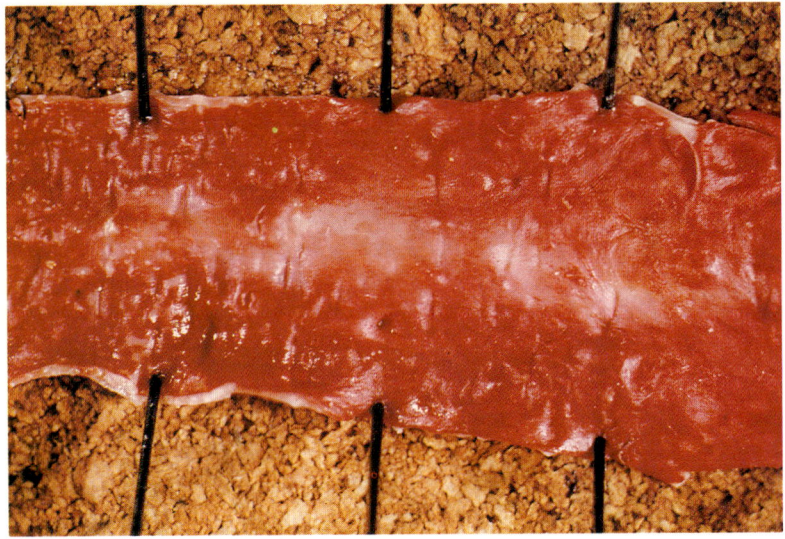

species or in unaffected areas of the intima in hypercholesterolaemic rabbits, is of the order of 8-10 times. Much of this increase is due to a marked increase in the intimal cell population. Many of the cells are large with a distinctly 'foamy' cytoplasm (Figure 1.27); their genesis is not ascertainable on light microscopy. Staining frozen sections with Sudan III and IV shows these foamy cells to be sudanophilic, and examination of unstained frozen sections under polarized light reveals large amounts of anisotropic intracellular material, indicating the presence of cholesterol. In lesions from older animals, some degree of necrosis is seen in the intima, and the basal and mid-portions of many of the plaques become virtually acellular with some focal dystrophic calcification.

Using transmission EM, the fine structure of endothelial cells in the affected area appears relatively normal, although occasional cells are vacuolated. In some areas, adjacent endothelial cells become separated from each other by large lipid-laden cells with ruffled plasma membranes and occasional intracytoplasmic myelin figures. Many researchers have reported similar appearances in a variety of species with hypercholesterolaemia induced by diet, regarding them as macrophages which have entered the artery wall from the blood, endocytosed lipid within the intima and are in the process of emigrating from the vessel wall back into the bloodstream. Definite identification of these cells as monocyte/macrophages is, as with the cell population of lesions in man, best carried out using monoclonal antibodies raised against various surface markers of the macrophage.

While it is almost certain that the macrophage constitutes an important part of the foam cell population in both experimentally induced and spontaneous atherosclerotic lesions, the intimal smooth muscle cell is also present in significant numbers. When the degree of distortion induced by lipid-loading is

Figure 1.27
Histological section through a fatty streak in a four-month-old hyperlipidaemic rabbit (St Thomas' Hospital strain). The intima is markedly thickened due to the presence of numerous large 'foam cells'.

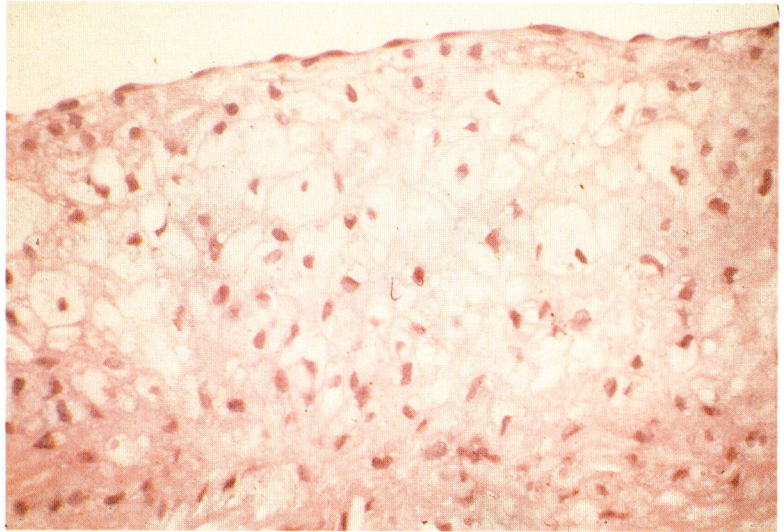

not too great, these cells can be recognized using EM by their elongated profiles, the presence of so-called 'dense bodies' at their periphery and evidence of basal lamina formation. The acellular areas at the base of the lesions show the presence of abundant extracellular lipid, mostly in the form of cholesterol 'clefts', and fragmented elastic fibres.

The use of SEM to examine vessels fixed by perfusion at physiological pressures shows surface ultrastructural changes in the youngest (10 weeks) affected animals examined so far. In many areas, the normally smooth and flat endothelial surface is interrupted by localized swellings where the cells appear to be stretched over subendothelial 'humps'. The concept that these subendothelial masses are accumulations of foam cells is supported by the finding in the aortas of animals more than four months old of focal defects in the endothelial lining from which aggregates of large cells with extensively ruffled plasma membranes protrude (Figure 1.28). These cells appear to be activated macrophages and are believed, as previously stated, to be emigrating from the subendothelial tissues into the blood. Cells with identical surface appearances are seen adhering to the luminal plasma membranes of endothelial cells in areas where there are no subendothelial swellings and, indeed, can be seen in relation to the intimal surfaces of human coronary artery lesions.

Cigarette-smoking and atherosclerosis
Heavy cigarette-smoking is strongly associated with CHD and peripheral vascular disease (177,196,197). Doll has estimated that the removal of the 'cigarette-smoke factor' may result in a 25% reduction in the current mortality from CHD. Even the passive exposure of non-smokers to cigarette smoke may increase the risk of CHD (198). In 1972, data from a prospective study by Hammond (199) showed that men aged between 40

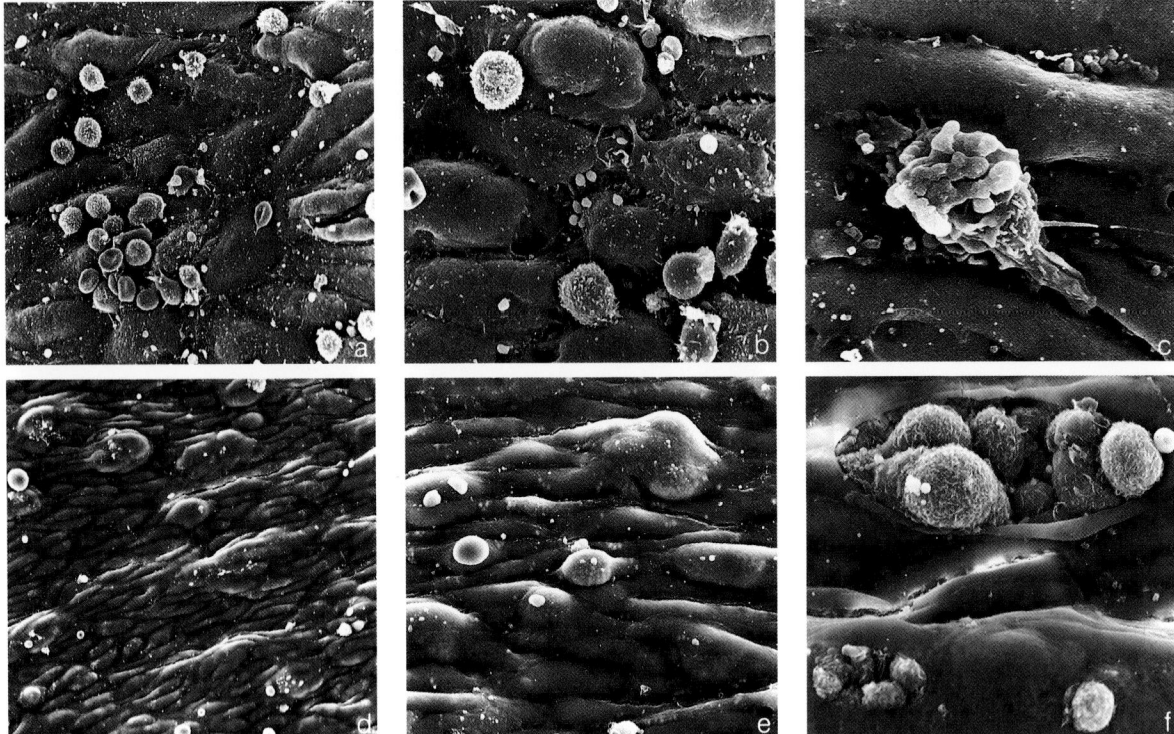

Figure 1.28
Scanning EMs of the aorta from a four-month-old hyperlipidaemic rabbit (St Thomas' Hospital strain): (a) large numbers of white cells are seen adhering to the endothelial surface; (b) high power view reveals many cells with the ruffled plasma membrane indicative of a monocyte/macrophage; (c) higher power view of a macrophage adherent to intact endothelium; (d) these hump-like protuberances on the intimal surface are subendothelial aggregates of macrophages, the expression of the next stage of fatty-streak formation. The endothelium is still intact; (e) high power view of fatty-streak formation reveals many of the endothelial cells to contain subendothelial lipid as punctate opacities; (f) higher power view shows focal cratered defects in the aortic endothelium, each occupied by an aggregate of ruffled macrophages.

and 49 years who smoked more than 40 cigarettes a day had a five-fold greater risk of dying from CHD than age-matched non-smokers. British data (200) indicated that, in men aged 45 to 54 years, smoking more than 15 cigarettes a day trebles the risk of dying from ischaemic heart disease, and similar results have been obtained in Framingham (201) and in Albany (202). In the Framingham study, all manifestations of myocardial underperfusion were increased, particularly myocardial infarction and sudden death; risk appeared to be more closely correlated with the number of cigarettes smoked daily rather than to duration of the habit. These data suggest that increased risk of major clinical events is mediated by mechanisms other than or in addition to a simple increase in the extent and severity of atherosclerosis (203), especially as the risk of CHD decreases in people who cease cigarette-smoking (204).

That cigarette-smoking has an effect on atherosclerosis was supported by results from a retrospective necropsy survey (205) in which smoking histories were obtained from relatives of deceased patients to evaluate the strength of the association between cigarette-smoking and atherosclerosis in 1320 males aged between 25 and 64 years. Atherosclerosis in the aorta and coronary arteries was greatest in heavy smokers and least in non-smokers. Other necropsy studies have yielded similar results (202,206-208), and the increase in atherosclerosis was primarily manifest as an increase in raised fibrolipid plaques (209).

Cigarette smoke-related endothelial changes

Well-defined ultrastructural changes in arterial endothelium as a result of exposure to cigarette smoke have been described by Asmussen (210-215) and Asmussen and Kjeldsen (216), who compared the morphological features of endothelium in umbilical vessels from the cords of infants born to either 'smoking' or 'non-smoking' mothers, and in uterine arteries in hysterectomy specimens from women who smoked (217). Umbilical artery endothelial cells from infants born to smoking mothers showed swelling and apparent contraction, and numerous blebs were seen in the luminal plasma membrane on SEM. On transmission EM, the endothelial cells were oedematous with marked dilatation of the cisternae and an increase in mitochondria. Oedema of the subendothelial space was a constant feature as was an increase in the thickness of the basement membrane.

Animal studies have shown that both acute and subacute exposure to cigarette smoke results in striking morphological changes in aortic endothelium in rabbits (218) and rats (219-221). In Pittilo's study, a single exposure to the fresh smoke of four cigarettes (diluted 1:3) resulted in a consistent pattern of changes in the luminal surface membrane in which blebs and the formation of microvillus-like projections was a constant feature (Figure 1.29). These alterations were confirmed on EMs which also revealed an increase in the number and size of plasmalemmal vesicles, which may be indicative of an increase in endothelial permeability.

The follow-up report of the Royal College of Physicians on smoking states:

"We still do not know what components of cigarette smoke

Figure 1.29
Scanning EM of rat aortic endothelium following exposure to graded doses of cigarette smoke. Note the presence of numerous small bleb-like protrusions on the luminal membrane.

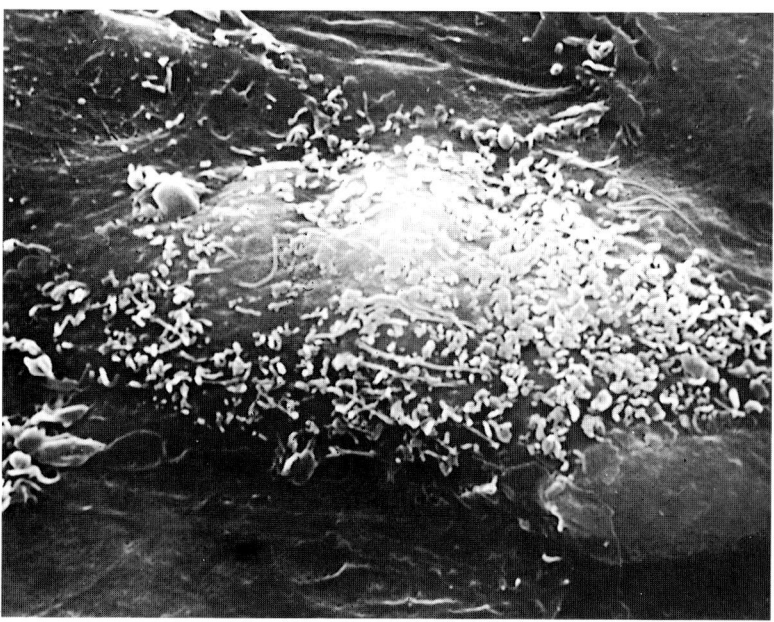

are responsible for the increased risk of cardiovascular disease."

The situation is much the same with regard to these morphological findings. Subacute exposure to nicotine (222,223) produces some morphological change in endothelium, but this is said to be less than that associated with exposure to whole smoke. Booyse and co-workers (224) were able to produce changes in cultured endothelium only with nicotine concentrations in excess of 10^{-4} M.

Changes in platelet – vessel wall interaction associated with exposure to cigarette smoke

In addition to changes in endothelial morphology as described in the aortas of animals exposed to cigarette smoke, microthrombi have been reported in such aortas most frequently in areas of low wall shear rate proximal to the ostia of the intercostal branches (219,221) (Figure 1.30). Such platelet adhesion appears to arise without detectable loss of endothelial cells from the underlying intima. In similarly treated animals, Pittilo and colleagues observed a marked decline in the ability of rings of aortic tissue to release the stable metabolite of prostacyclin (PGI_2), and similar effects on arterial prostanoid metabolism have been reported by other workers (225,226). Madsen and Dyerberg (227) found that smoking two high-nicotine-containing cigarettes by habitual smokers caused a significant reduction in bleeding time which could be prevented by aspirin. This was attributed to decreased production of PGI_2. Belch and colleagues (228) showed that cigarette smokers had higher plasma fibrinogen, lower plasminogen and plasminogen activator concentrations, and higher plasma viscosity. The changes observed in smokers after smoking three cigarettes were an increase in the rate of platelet aggregation to ADP, an increase in alpha-2-macroglobulin and an increase in

Figure 1.30
Scanning EM of rat aorta following exposure to graded doses of cigarette smoke showing the proximal part of the ostium. Adherent and aggregated platelets are seen on an apparently intact endothelial surface.

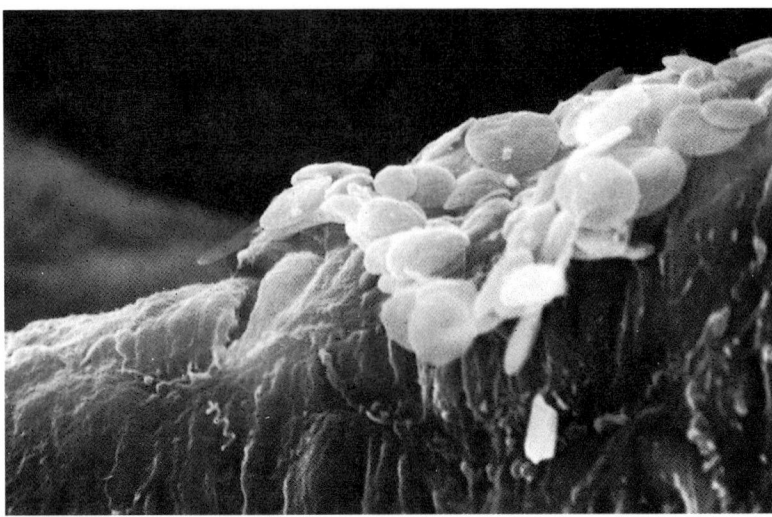

Factor VIII:RAG. Plasma viscosity was decreased as was red cell deformation. These results suggest that cigarette-smoking affects the platelet-coagulation axis and, thus, may contribute to increased risk for atherosclerosis-related events.

Cigarette smoke-related effects on arterial endothelium cannot be directly studied in man, but an increase in the number of circulating endothelial cells in human volunteers after cigarette-smoking has been observed (229-231).

Pittilo (232) devised an ex-vivo model to investigate the possible cytotoxicity of cigarette smoke and its metabolites. Cultured mesothelial cells derived from human omentum were exposed to plasma taken before and shortly after cigarette-smoking. Cultures exposed to the pre-smoking sample showed no significant morphological changes on SEM, while those treated with post-smoking plasma samples showed severe blebbing (as seen *in vivo*), contraction and detachment from the underlying surface.

Thus, cigarette-smoking is associated with morphological and functional alterations in endothelium. The mechanisms are not yet fully understood, although tobacco glycoprotein, produced from flue-cured tobacco leaves, is mitogenic for bovine arterial smooth muscle cells (233).

Recently, a study (234) of the effects of cigarette-smoking on specific haemostatic factors demonstrated associations between high levels of Factor VII_c and plasma fibrinogen concentration, which are also risk factors for CHD. The duration of smoking is a determinant of plasma fibrinogen levels. When smoking is discontinued, fibrinogen levels decrease, reaching that of non-smokers after five years. In prospective data, changes in smoking habits lead to changes of approximately 0.15 g/l in plasma fibrinogen, which may lower or raise the risk of CHD by approximately 20%.

Diabetes mellitus and atherosclerosis

Diabetes, atherosclerosis and hyperlipidaemia are all closely linked (235). Atherosclerosis-related disease, especially CHD, is a major complication of both insulin-dependent and non-insulin-dependent diabetes, such arterial disease now accounting for more than 70% of all deaths from both forms of diabetes (235). A recent report suggests that by the age of 50 years, one-third of insulin-dependent diabetics will have died from atherosclerosis-related disease, a large proportion of whom will have had coincident renal disease (236). The degree of increased risk is even higher in diabetic women, who appear to lose their relative immunity from atherosclerosis-related vascular disease during their reproductive years. It appears, however, that if diabetes is to operate fully as a risk factor, a specific 'background' level of atherosclerosis is required, as the presence of diabetes in low-risk populations does not increase the risk of CHD.

Atherosclerosis in diabetics and non-diabetics
Ideally, the effects of diabetes on the arterial tree should be examined in deceased subjects who, apart from the presence or absence of diabetes, are similar in other respects. It is difficult, however, to assemble a large enough number of cases which meet this criterion. In the IAP study, a compromise was adopted. Two studies were carried out: In the first, all patients with diabetes were compared with those without; in the second, all other conditions putatively related to atherosclerosis (for example, hypertension) were eliminated from the sample (237). When the intimal surface involvement by fatty streaks was analyzed, no significant differences were found between the abdominal aortas of diabetics and non-diabetics. Regarding aortic fibrolipid plaques, however, there was an increased incidence in diabetics, although this was not always significant. The coronary arteries in diabetics showed an increase in both the extent of involvement by fatty streaks and by fibrolipid plaques. Similar morphological data have been reported in a necropsy study of the effects of diabetes on Japanese-American men (238).

Why are diabetics more at risk for arterial disease?
Factors commonly recognized as increasing the risk of arterial disease, such as hypercholesterolaemia, high blood pressure and cigarette-smoking, are equally and, in some cases, more prevalent in diabetics than in non-diabetics. In the Multiple Risk Factor Intervention Trial (MRFIT), these three factors were as strongly related to CHD in the diabetic as in the non-diabetic portion of the large sample followed-up for six years. However:

> For each risk factor and at every level of risk, the mortality from CHD among diabetics was three-fold higher than that in non-diabetics (239).

This suggests that risk factors other than the above-mentioned may be operative in diabetics, one of which may be hyperinsulinaemia that, indeed, appears to be a risk factor for CHD in both diabetics and non-diabetics (240).

Blood pressure
As with diabetes mellitus, elevated blood pressure is an important risk factor for CHD in those countries where atherosclerosis-related disease is common (Figure 1.31). In low-risk populations, such as those in developing countries, hypertension is not uncommon and is associated with haemorrhagic stroke and renal failure, but not with an increased risk of CHD. As Shaper (169) has pointed out, there are difficul-

ties in defining raised blood pressure. In the British Regional Heart Study, a two-fold increase in the risk of CHD was evident with a systolic blood pressure over 148 mmHg, and diastolic pressures over 93 mmHg were associated with a greater than two-fold risk. Diastolic BP levels between 72 to 92 mmHg were also associated with a significantly increased risk of CHD when compared with those below 72 mmHg. In the Framingham study, a blood pressure higher than 160/95 mmHg was regarded as hypertensive and carried a two-fold increase in risk of CHD.

In the IAP study, Robertson and Strong (237) showed that hypertension was associated with an increase in the extent of fatty streaks both in the abdominal aorta and coronary arteries. As regards fibrolipid plaques, there was a statistically significant difference between hypertensive and normotensive subjects at all ages, in both sexes, and in both aorta and coronary arteries. These data indicate that elevated blood pressure in the systemic circulation is associated with an increased degree of atherogenesis and are supported by the results of many animal studies showing that a combination of hyperlipidaemia and elevated blood pressure levels results in more extensive arterial lesions than hyperlipidaemia alone. The mechanism(s) by which hypertension produces this incremental ef-

Figure 1.31
Incremental effects of risk factors of CHD (hypertension, hyperlipidaemia and cigarette-smoking) on mortality in white males (aged 35 to 57 years) taking part in US MRFIT study. From Mitchell, 1984, with permission.

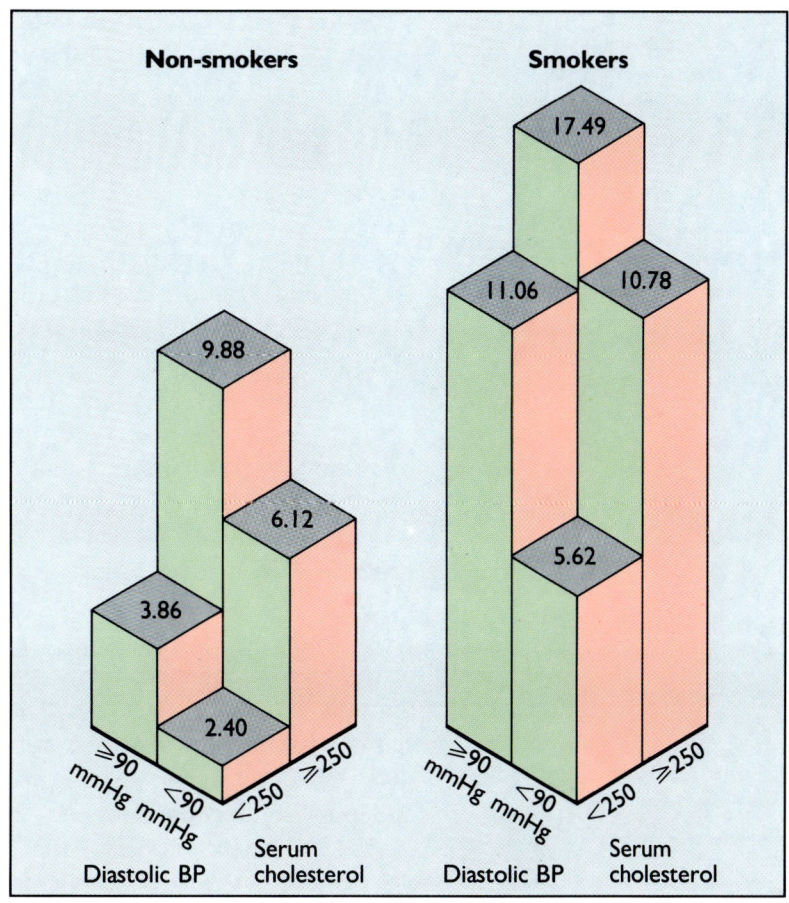

fect on atherogenesis is not known. In addition, despite the evidence that hypertension is a risk factor for both atherosclerosis and CHD, it is disappointing that, in the various primary prevention trials carried out in hypertensives, the differences in myocardial infarction rates between treatment and control groups were small and not significant overall (241).

Inhibition and regression of atherosclerosis
Inhibition of lesion development
The term 'inhibition' implies prevention or postponement of the development of atherosclerotic lesions, and the significant differences in the extent and severity of atherosclerosis between populations may be sufficient evidence that such inhibition does occur. Animals with genetically determined hyperlipidaemias are good models of inhibition, especially if this is mediated through drugs. Carew and colleagues (155) and Kita and co-workers (156) were the first to show that fatty-streak development (in the WWHL rabbit) could be significantly reduced. Control rabbits in the former study had total plasma cholesterol levels of 761 ±29 mg/dl. This was reduced to 671 ±23 mg/dl after treatment with probucol and, with lovastatin (an HMG-CoA-reductase inhibitor) at a low dosage (2 mg/kg/day), plasma cholesterol levels fell to 618 ±21 mg/dl. The extent of lesions in the aorta (expressed as a percentage of the surface area involved) was 40.6 ±5.1% in the untreated controls, 27.5 ±4.6% in animals receiving lovastatin, and 14.3 ±2.1% in those receiving probucol. In addition to demonstrating that lesion development could be reduced with hypolipidaemic agents, the effect of probucol suggests that its antioxidant properties may also be very important. The results obtained in the study by Kita and colleagues were even more striking in terms of inhibition of lesion development, although probucol appeared to produce a greater decrease in plasma cholesterol concentrations.

Lovastatin was also used in another primary prevention study of atherosclerosis (241) in the St Thomas' Hospital rabbit, a model for familial combined hyperlipidaemia (15,195). The animals were divided into two groups and matched for weight, plasma cholesterol and plasma triglyceride levels. One group received lovastatin at a dose of 12 mg/kg/day and the other served as a control. Plasma lipids were measured at two-week intervals, and two animals from each group were killed at the ages of four, six, 7.5, 8.5 and 10.5 months. The treated animals showed a 60% decrease in plasma cholesterol compared with the controls; this was due to reduced levels of LDL and IDL cholesterol. Concentrations of the other lipoprotein classes remained unchanged. The extent of fatty streaks (expressed as a percentage of the intimal surface area involved) was markedly reduced in the treated animals compared with the controls (Figures 1.32 & 1.33). Mean surface area involvement in the treated animals was 4.2 ±1.9% (range 0 – 16.2%) whereas, in the controls, the mean was 26.1 ±9.2% (range 0.3 – 85.7%). The intima:media ratio (measurements being taken for the whole aorta) in the controls was 0.421:1, and 0.120:1 in the treated rabbits. The extent of aortic disease was significantly related to the LDL-cholesterol concentration when adjusted for the age of the animals; the relationship with IDL-cholesterol concentrations was not significant when adjusted for age. Such studies are in themselves interesting and valuable as they emphasize the potential importance of LDL-cholesterol concentrations and of LDL oxidation in the genesis of atherosclerotic plaques as well as provide a model for the screening of 'antiatherogenic' (not necessarily hypolipidaemic) compounds.

One group of such compounds are the calcium antagonists. A number of studies have been carried out both in cholesterol-fed and in WHHL rabbits to assess the effects of calcium antagonists, such as diltiazem and nifedipine (242-251). The re-

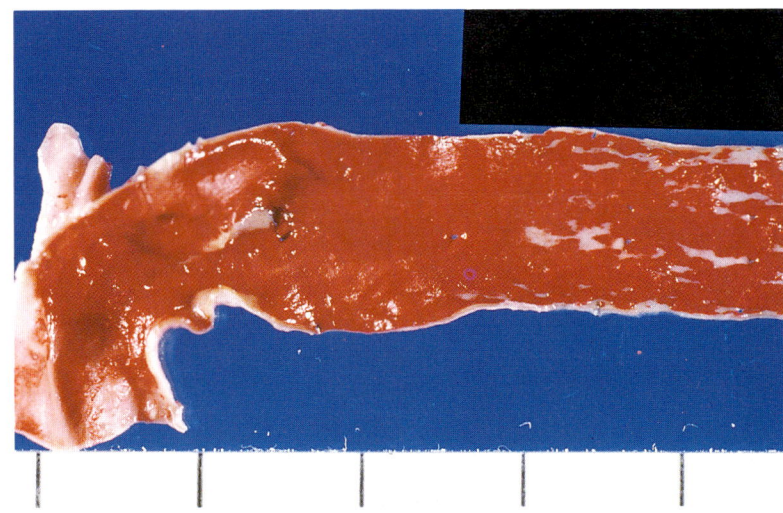

Figure 1.32
Post-mortem section of thoracic aorta from a 7.5-month-old hyperlipidaemic rabbit (St Thomas' Hospital strain) which had received a placebo since weaning. After treatment with a fat-soluble dye, virtually the whole of the intimal surface appears red, indicating lipid deposition.

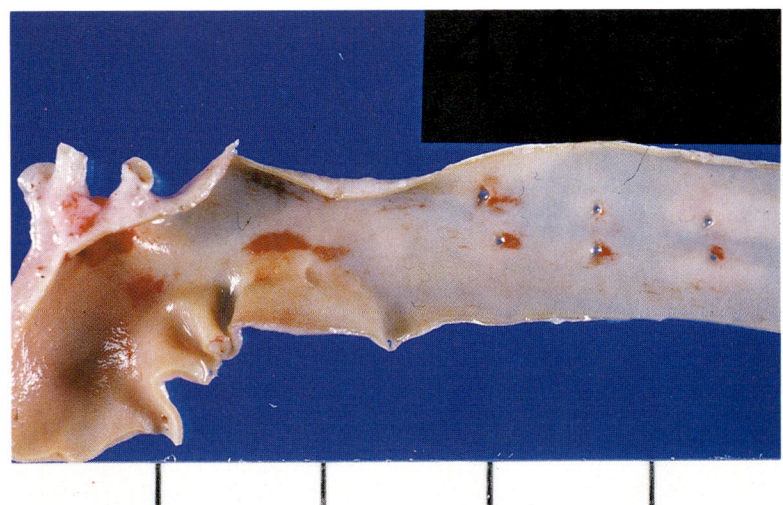

Figure 1.33
Post-mortem section of thoracic aorta of a 7.5-month-old hyperlipidaemic rabbit (St Thomas' Hospital strain) with the same plasma cholesterol concentration at weaning as the rabbit in Figure 1.32. This rabbit, however, had been given HMG-CoA reductase inhibitor at a dose of 12 mg/kg daily, which resulted in significant inhibition of lipid deposition.

sults have been conflicting. In some cases, there appears to have been inhibition of lesion development in cholesterol-fed animals, but not in those with genetically determined hyperlipidaemia. In a study of the effect of two calcium antagonists on the natural history of balloon-catheter lesions in the rat carotid artery, it was noted that inhibition of the usual post-injury smooth muscle cell proliferation was brought about by the compound isradipine (PN 200-110; 250). However, in the 'real-life' atherosclerotic situation, proliferation of smooth muscle and extracellular matrices constitute only part of the problem.

The effects of calcium antagonists have been studied at least once in man (251). A double-blind angiographic trial was carried out in patients with 'mild coronary artery disease'. Of the patients receiving placebo, 49% developed 118 new lesions *in toto* over a three-year period whereas 41% of the patients receiving nifedipine developed a total of 79 new lesions. However, no difference was seen between the placebo and treatment groups in the progression of existing lesions.

Regression of lesions

From the practical clinical point of view, of much greater importance is whether dietary and/or pharmacological manoeuvres can shrink established atherosclerotic plaques while increasing the dimensions of the arterial lumen and, if possible, the perfusion of the affected tissues. It is important to realize that a decrease within a population of the risk of ischaemic heart disease is not synonymous with lesion regression, as the extent and severity of wall disease may not be the only factor involved. There is evidence, albeit some of which is anecdotal, that such a decline in risk within a single population can occur. Most accounts of this phenomenon are related to wartime experiences (252-255). Necropsy studies carried out in Germany after World War I reportedly showed a decrease in the extent and severity of atherosclerotic lesions (253,256,257). There is, indeed, a considerable body of evidence from both man and experimental animals that reduction in the size and changes in the constituents of atherosclerotic lesions does occur (258-262).

In the words of Alexander Pope: *"The proper study of mankind is man."*

This dictum is equally applicable to the study of vascular diseases. Many difficulties obstruct evaluation of the extent and severity of atherosclerosis in life. At present, the only practical method for assessing the effect of any diet and/or drug regime on atherosclerotic lesions is sequential angiography; the introduction of non-invasive technology, such as nuclear magnetic resonance imaging of these lesions, could be of immense value (263). The use of sequential angiography for assessing the progression, regression or stability of a given lesion must be monitored with extreme care as there are many factors which may nullify the value of such studies (264). It must also be remembered that with angiography, it is the dimension and outline of the vascular lumen which are being delineated and not the atherosclerotic plaque itself (265).

Despite these reservations, many data have accrued, especially since the introduction of computerized image analysis of angiograms by Blankenhorn and colleagues (266,267). Resolution technology is now able to measure changes of 0.05 to 0.1 mm (268). In 1976, San Marco and co-workers (269) described a series of 42 patients in whom femoral arteriography had been performed before and after a year of treatment for hyperlipidaemia and other risk factors. After an average time of 15 months, angiographic improvement was found in six patients, stabilization in 16 patients and further progression of disease in another 16.

In the UK, the first randomized controlled trial of the effects of risk factor intervention on angiographic appearances in affected vessels was carried out in 24 hyperlipidaemic subjects complaining of intermittent claudication due to atherosclerosis of the femoral artery. The intervention group was treated with diet, advised to stop smoking if appropriate, and received cholestyramine, nicotinic acid or clofibrate for periods of 18 to 24 months (270). On angiographic assessment of 144 arterial segments from the intervention group and 154 segments from the control group, 6.9% and 17.3% of plaques respectively showed progression. The mean increase in plaque area per annum was 0.58 mm^2 in the intervention group and 1.72 mm^2 in the controls. Computerized image analysis showed a mean change in the 'edge irregularity index' of 0.019 in the intervention group and 0.047 in the controls. In this study, there was a significant correlation between the mean levels of LDL and the extent of progression of femoral artery atherosclerosis (r = 0.57).

In 1985, Arntzenius and colleagues (271) carried out an intervention study in Leiden in a group of 39 patients with stable angina in whom coronary angiography had demonstrated severe narrowing (more than 50%) in two major vessels. Intervention consisted of a two-year vegetarian diet that had a 2:1 ratio of polyunsaturated to saturated fatty acids and a cholesterol content of less than 100 mg/day. There was no control group, and the data were analyzed by relating angiographic progression or stability to mean lipid and lipoprotein levels during the study. Angiographic evidence of lesion progression was seen in 21 patients and no such progression in 18. Those showing lesion progression also had higher mean cholesterol concentrations and slightly lower plasma HDL-cholesterol concentrations than those in whom lesions did not progress. Changes in vessel diameter correlated positively with the ratio of mean total cholesterol:HDL cholesterol. In this study, however, there was no lesion regression as the result of treatment but, rather, an absence of progression.

The National Heart, Lung and Blood Institute conducted a five-year randomized controlled trial in 116 patients with angina whose mean plasma cholesterol concentration was 8.4 mmol/l (272). Approximately half of the sample had familial hypercholesterolaemia. Both the control and treatment groups were stabilized on a low-fat/low-cholesterol diet, then randomly allocated to receive either cholestyramine or placebo. Diet alone reduced the LDL cholesterol by 6% in both groups. After randomization, LDL cholesterol decreased by a further 5% in the placebo group and by 26% in the cholestyramine group. Coronary angiography was carried out before and after the five-year treatment period. Progression was found in 49% of the placebo group and in 32% of the treatment group. 'Definite lesion regression' was recorded in one of the 57 controls and in three of the 59 treated subjects. While all of the angiographic indices favoured the cholestyramine-treated subjects, the results did not achieve statistical significance although, when only lesions causing 50% or greater stenosis are considered, the progression rate was 12% in the treatment group compared to 33% in the controls. This result was significant ($p < 0.05$), but must be viewed with caution as this subgroup was not defined at the beginning of the study.

The most convincing study of the effect of lipid-lowering treatment on the evolution of coronary artery atherosclerosis is CLAS (Cholesterol-Lowering Atherosclerosis Study). This was described by Blankenhorn and colleagues in 1987 (273). The participants were 162 non-smoking men who had undergone coronary artery-bypass grafting. Total plasma cholesterol concentrations at entry ranged from 4.8 to 9.1 mmol/l with a mean of 6.35 mmol/l. Coronary, carotid and femoral artery angiograms were obtained at baseline and two years later. The participants were randomized to either active treatment (colestipol 30 g/day plus nicotinic acid 3 to 12 g/day) or to control. Both treatment and control groups received appropriate dietary advice. After two years of treatment, there was a 26% reduction in total plasma cholesterol, a 43% reduction in LDL cholesterol and a 37% elevation in HDL cholesterol. This was associated with a significant reduction in the average number of progressive lesions per subject ($p < 0.03$) and in the percentage of subjects with new lesions ($p < 0.04$) in either the 'native' coronary arteries or bypass grafts. Progression and/or regression of atherosclerosis, as determined from the angiographic data, were expressed as global score changes. On this basis, regression was recorded in 2.4% of the controls and 16.2% of the treatment group. No change was noted in 36.6% of the controls and in 45% of the treatment group, and progression occurred in 61% of the controls and in 38.8% of the treatment group.

The overall conclusion to be drawn from these studies is that in man and in a number of animal models, reduction of plasma cholesterol concentrations by a variety of means may influence the natural history of atherosclerotic lesions. However, whether such treatment will produce a similar reduction in the frequency of major clinical events or in the mortality from ischaemic heart disease is less certain. The outlook, however, is encouraging.

References

1. Marchand F. Über arteriosklerose. *Verhandlung der Kongres für innere Medizin* 1904; **21**: 23-59.

2. Shattock SG. A report upon the pathological condition of the aorta of King Menephthah, traditionally regarded as the Pharoah of the Exodus. *Proc Roy Soc Med Path* 1909; **2**: 122-7.

3. Ruffer MA. On arterial lesions found in Egyptian mummies. *J Pathol Bacteriol* 1911; **15**: 453-62.

4. Sandison AT. Diseases of the ancient world. In: Anthony PP, MacSween RNM, eds. *Recent Advances in Pathology, Volume 11*. Edinburgh: Churchill Livingstone, 1981: 1-18.

5. Morgan AD. *The Pathogenesis of Coronary Occlusion*. Oxford: Blackwell, 1956.

6. Long ER. Development of our knowledge of arteriosclerosis. In: Blumenthal HT, ed. *Cowdry's Arteriosclerosis*. Springfield, Charles C Thomas; 1967: 5-20.

7. Crawford T. Some aspects of the pathology of atherosclerosis. *Proc Roy Soc Med* 1960; **53**: 62-9.

8. Davies MJ, Thomas AC. Pathological basis and microanatomy of occlusive thrombus formation in human coronary arteries. In: Born GVR, Vane JR, eds. *Interactions Between Platelets and Vessel Walls*. London: Roy Soc 1981; 9-12.

9. Falk E. Plaque rupture with severe pre-existing stenosis precipitating coronary thrombosis: Characteristics of coronary atherosclerotic plaques underlying fatal occlusive thrombi. *Br Heart J* 1983; **50**: 127-34.

10. Davies MJ, Thomas AC. Thrombosis in acute coronary artery lesions in sudden ischaemic death. *N Engl J Med* 1984; **310**: 1137-40.

11. Haust MD. The morphogenesis and fate of potential and early atherosclerotic lesions in man. *Hum Pathol* 1971; **2**: 1-30.

12. Gerrity RG, Naito HK, Richardson M, Schwartz CJ. Dietary induced atherogenesis in swine: Morphology of the intima in prelesion stages. *Am J Pathol* 1979; **95**: 775.

13. Faggiotto A, Ross R. Studies of hypercholesterolemia in the non-human primate. II. Fatty streak conversion to fibrous plaque. *Arteriosclerosis* 1984; **4**: 341.

14. Rosenfeld ME, Tsukada T, Gown AM, Ross R. Fatty streak initiation in Watanabe heritable hyperlipemic and comparable hypercholesterolemic fat-fed rabbits.

Arteriosclerosis 1987; **7**: 9-23.

15. Seddon AM, Woolf N, LaVille A, et al. Hereditary hyperlipidaemia and atherosclerosis in the rabbit due to over-production of lipoproteins. II. Preliminary report of arterial pathology. *Arteriosclerosis* 1987; **7**: 113-24.

16. Taylor RG, Lewis JC. Endothelial cell proliferation and monocyte adhesion to atherosclerotic lesions of white Carneau pigeons. *Am J Pathol* 1986; **125**: 152-60.

17. Schwartz CJ, Ardlie NG, Carter RF, Paterson JC. Gross aortic sudanophilia and hemosiderin deposition. A study on infants, children and young adults. *Arch Pathol* 1967; **83**: 325-32.

18. Caro CG, Fitzgerald JM, Schroter RC. Arterial wall shear and distribution of early atheroma in man. *Nature* 1969; **223**: 1159-60.

19. Caro CG, Fitzgerald JM, Schroter RC. Atheroma and arterial wall shear. Observation, correlation and proposal of a shear dependent mass transfer mechanism for atherogenesis. *Proc Roy Soc Lond* 1971; **177**: 109-59.

20. Chien S. Significance of macrorheology and microrheology in atherogenesis. *Ann NY Acad Sci* 1976; **275**: 10-27.

21. Fowler S. Characterization of foam cells in experimental atherosclerosis. In: *Proc. 5th Paavo Nurmi Symposium: Thrombosis and Blood Vessel Wall Interaction in Coronary Heart Disease*. Acta Med Scand (Suppl) 1980; **642**: 151-8.

22. Mitchinson MJ. Macrophages, oxidised lipids and atherosclerosis. *Med Hypoth* 1983; **12**: 171-8.

23. Klurfeld DM. Identification of foam cells in human atherosclerotic lesions as macrophages using monoclonal antibodies. *Arch Pathol Lab Med* 1985; **109**: 445-9.

24. Mitchinson MJ, Ball RY. Macrophages and atherogenesis. *Lancet* 1987; **ii**: 146-9.

25. Davies MJ, Woolf N, Rowles PM, Pepper J. Morphology of the endothelium over atherosclerotic plaques in human coronary arteries. *Br Heart J* 1988; **60**: 459-64.

26. McGill HC Jr. The lesion. In: Schettler G, Weizel A, eds. *Atherosclerosis III. Proc Third Int Symposium*. Berlin: Springer-Verlag, 1974; 27-38.

27. Faggiotto A, Ross R, Harker L. Studies of hypercholesterolemia in the nonhuman primate. I. Changes that lead to fatty streak

formation. *Arteriosclerosis* 1984; **4**: 323.

28. Restrepo C, Tracy RE. Variation in human aortic fatty streaks among geographic locations. *Atherosclerosis* 1975; **21**: 179-93.

29. Wolkoff K. Über die histologische structur der coronärarterien des menschlichen Herzens. *Virchows Arch Pathol Anat* 1923; **241-3**: 42-58.

30. Smith EB. Development of the atheromatous lesion. In: Wolf S, Werthessen NT, eds. *The Smooth Muscle of the Artery. Adv Exp Med Biol* 1975; **57**; 254-60.

31. More RM, Haust MD. Role of mural fibrin thrombi in genesis of arteriosclerotic plaques. *Arch Pathol* 1957; **63**: 612-20.

32. Movat H, Haust MD, More RH. The morphological elements in the early lesion of atherosclerosis. *Am J Pathol* 1959; **35**: 93-101.

33. Woolf N. The distribution of fibrin within the aortic intima: An immunohistochemical study. *Am J Pathol* 1961; **39**: 521-32.

34. Smith EB. Atherosclerotic lesions – an overview. In: Crepaldi G, Gotto AM, Manzato E, Baggio, eds. *Atherosclerosis VIII*. Amsterdam, New York, Oxford: Excerpta Medica, 1989; 13-19.

35. Smith EB. Fibrinogen and fibrin degradation products in relation to atherosclerosis. *Clin Haematol* 1986; **15**: 355.

36. Thompson WD, McGuigan CJ, Snyder C, Keen GA, Smith EB. Mitogenic activity in human atherosclerotic lesions. *Atherosclerosis* 1987; **66**: 85-93.

37. Tejada C, Strong JP, Montenegro MR, Restrepo C, Solberg LA. Distribution of aortic and coronary atherosclerosis by geographic location, race and sex. *Lab Invest* 1968; **18**: 509-26.

38. Strong JP, Solberg LA, Restrepo C. Atherosclerosis in persons with coronary heart disease. *Lab Invest* 1968; **18**: 527-37.

39. Deupree RH, Fields RI, McMahan CA, Strong JP. Atherosclerotic lesions and coronary heart disease. Key relationships in necropsied cases. *Lab Invest* 1973; **28**: 252-62.

40. Ross R, Wight TN, Strandness E, Thiel B. Human atherosclerosis. I. Cell constitution and characterization of advanced lesions of the superficial femoral artery. *Am J Pathol* 1984; **114**: 79-93.

41. Adams CWM, Bayliss OB. The relationship between diffuse intimal thickness, medial enzyme failure and intimal lipid deposit in various human arteries. *J Ath Rev* 1969; **10**: 327-39.

42. Mitchell JRA, Schwartz CJ. The planometric assessment of aortic disease severity. In: *Arterial Disease*: Oxford; Blackwell Scientific Publications, 1965: 386-96.

43. Albutt C. *Diseases of the arteries, including Angina Pectoris.* London: MacMillan, 1915: 468.

44. Schwartz CJ, Mitchell JRA. Cellular infiltration of human arterial adventitia associated with atheromatous plaques. *Circulation* 1962; **26**: 73.

45. Parums D, Mitchinson MJ. Demonstration of immunoglobulin in the neighbourhood of advanced atherosclerotic plaques. *Atherosclerosis* 1981; **38**: 211-6.

46. Duguid JB. Thrombosis as a factor in the pathogenesis of coronary atherosclerosis. *J Pathol Bacteriol* 1946; **58**: 207-12.

47. Duguid JB. Thrombosis as a factor in the pathogenesis of aortic atherosclerosis. *J Pathol Bacteriol* 1948; **60**: 57-61.

48. Duguid JB. *The Dynamics of Atherosclerosis.* Aberdeen: Aberdeen University Press, 1976: 44-9.

49. Rokitansky K Von. *Handbuch der Pathologisches Anatomie, Volume 2.* Braunmuller and Seidel, 1844.

50. Heard BE. An experimental study of thickening of the pulmonary arteries of rabbits produced by organisation of fibrin. *J Pathol Bacteriol* 1949; **64**: 13-9.

51. Crawford T, Levene CI. Incorporation of fibrin in the aortic intima. *J Pathol Bacteriol* 1952; **64**: 523-8.

52. Woolf N, Crawford T. Fatty streaks in aortic intima studied by an immunohistochemical technique. *J Pathol Bacteriol* 1960; **80**: 405-8.

53. Wyllie JC, More RH, Haust MD. Demonstration of fibrin in yellow aortic streaks by the fluorescent antibody technique. *J Pathol Bacteriol* 1964. **88**: 335-8.

54. Haust MD, Wyllie JC, More RH. Electron microscopy of fibrin in human atherosclerotic lesions. Immunohistochemical and morphological identification. *Exp Mol Pathol* 1965; **4**: 205-16.

55. Kao VCY, Wissler RW. A study of the immunochemical localization of serum lipoproteins and other plasma proteins in human atherosclerotic lesions. *Exp Mol Pathol* 1965; **4**: 465-79.

56. Smith EB, Massie IB, Alexander KM. Insoluble 'fibrin' in human aortic intima. Quantitative studies on the relationship between insoluble 'fibrin', soluble fibrinogen and low density lipoprotein. *Atherosclerosis* 1976; **23**: 19-39.

57. Carstairs KC. The identification of platelets and platelet antigens in tissue sections. *J Pathol Bacteriol* 1965; **90**: 225-31.

58. Woolf N, Carstairs KC. The survival time of platelets in experimental mural thrombi. *J Pathol* 1969; **97** 595-601.

59. Hudson J, McCaughey WTE. Mural thrombosis and atherogenesis in coronary arteries and aorta. *Atherosclerosis* 1974; **19**: 543-53.

60. Chandler AB, Terrell Pope J. Arterial thrombosis in atherogenesis. In: Hautvast JGAJ, Hermus RJJ, van der Haar F (eds). *Blood and Arterial Wall in Atherogenesis and Arterial Thrombosis*: Leiden, Brill. Iifma Scientific Symposium No. 4; 111-118.

61. Woolf N, Sacks MI, Davies MJ. Aortic plaque morphology in relation to coronary artery disease. *Am J Pathol* 1969; **57**: 187-97.

62. Meade TW, North WRS, Chakrabarti R, et al. Haemostatic function and cardiovascular death: early results of a prospective study. *Lancet* 1980; **i**: 1050-4.

63. Meade TW. Thrombogenic factors. In: Olsson AG, ed. *Atherosclerosis: Biology and Clinical Science.* Edinburgh, London, Melbourne, New York: Churchill Livingstone, 1987: 453-5.

64. Campbell GR, Campbell JH. Smooth muscle cells. In: Olsson AG, ed. *Atherosclerosis: Biology and Clinical Science.* Edinburgh, London, Melbourne, New York; Churchill Livingstone, 1987: 453-5.

65. Burke JM, Ross R. Synthesis of connective tissue macromolecules by smooth muscle. *Int Rev Connect Tissue Res* 1979; **8**: 119-57.

66. Narayanan AS, Sandberg LE, Ross R, Layman DL. The smooth muscle cell. III. Elastin synthesis in arterial smooth muscle cell culture. *J Cell Biol* 1976; **68**: 411-9.

67. Ross R. Platelets, smooth muscle proliferation and atherosclerosis. *Acta Med Scand* 1980; **642 (Suppl)**: 49-54.

68. Ross R. The smooth muscle cell in connective tissue metabolism and atherosclerosis. In: Kulonen E, ed. *Proc Sigrid Juselius Foundation Symposium, Turku, Finland; The Biology of the Fibroblast.* London: Academic Press, 1973; 623-36.

69. McCullagh KE, Balian G. Collagen characterization and cell transformation in human atherosclerosis. *Nature* 1975; **258**: 73-5.

70. Ross R, Glomset J, Kariya B, Harker L. A platelet-dependent serum factor that stimulates the proliferation of arterial smooth muscle cells in vitro. *Proc Nat'l Acad Sci USA* 1974; **71**: 1207.

71. Rutherford RB, Ross R. Platelet factors stimulate fibroblasts and smooth muscle cells quiescent in plasma serum to proliferate. *J Cell Biol* 1976; **69**: 196-200.

72. Ross R, Glomset J, Harker L. Response to injury and atherogenesis. *Am J Pathol* 1977. **86**: 675-84.

73. Ross R, Harker L. Platelets, endothelium and smooth muscle cells in atherosclerosis. In: Day HJ, Molony BA, Nishizawa EE, Rynbarth RH, eds. *Thrombosis: Animal and Clinical Models.* New York: Plenum Press, 1978: 125-44.

74. Ross R. The pathogenesis of atherosclerosis – an update. *N Engl J Med* 1986; **314**: 488-501.

75. Ross R. Cellular interactions in atherosclerosis – the role of growth factors. In: Crepaldi G, Gotto AM, Manzato E, Baggio G, eds. *Atherosclerosis VIII.* Amsterdam, New York, Oxford, 1989: Excerpta Medica, 13-19.

76. Betzholtz C, Johnsson A, Aildin C-H, et al. c-DNA and chromosomal localization of human platelet derived growth factor A-gene and its expression in tumour cell lines. *Nature* 1986; **320**: 695-9.

77. Swan DC, McBride DW, Robbins KC, Keithley DA, Reddy EP, Aaronson SA. Chromosomal mapping of the simian sarcoma virus onc-gene analogue in human cells. *Proc Nat'l Acad Sci* 1982; **79**: 4691-5.

78. Waterfield MD, Scrace GT, Whittle H, et al. Platelet-derived growth factor is structurally related to the putative transforming protein p28^{v-sis} of simian sarcoma virus. *Nature* 1983; **304**: 35-9.

79. Doolittle RF, Hunkapiller MW, Hood LE, et al. Simian sarcoma virus oncogene, v-sis, is derived from the gene (or genes) encoding a platelet-derived growth factor. *Science* 1983; **221**: 275-7.

80. Sporn MB, Roberts AB. Autocrine growth factors in cancer. *Nature* 1985; **313**: 745.

81. Habernicht AJR, Glomset JA, King WC, Nist C, Mitchell CD, Ross R. Early changes in phosphatidylinositol and arachidonic acid metabolism in quiescent Swiss 3T3 cells stimulated to divide by platelet-derived growth factor. *J Biol Chem* 1981; **256**: 12329-35.

82. Shier WT, Durkin JP. Role of stimulation of arachidonic acid release in the proliferative response of 3T3 mouse fibroblasts to platelet-derived growth factor. *J Cell Physiol* 1982; **112**: 171-81.

83. Habernicht AJR, Georig M, Grulich J, et al. Human platelet-derived growth factor stimulates prostaglandin synthesis by activation and by rapid de novo synthesis of cyclooxygenase. *J Clin Invest* 1985; **75**: 1381-7.

84. Waterfield MD. The role of growth factors in cancer. In: Franks LM, Teich N, eds. *Introduction to the Cellular and Molecular Biology of Cancer.* Oxford: Oxford University Press, 1986; 251-76.

85. Berridge JL, Irvine RF. Inositol triphosphate, a novel second messenger in cellular signal transduction. *Nature* 1984; **312**: 315-21.

86. Nemeth GG, Bolander ME, Martin GR. Growth factors and their role in wound and fracture healing. In: Hurst T, ed. *Growth Factors and Other Aspects of Wound Healing; Biological and Clinical Implications.* New

York: Alan R Liss, 1988; 1-18.

87. Gadjusek CM, DiCorleto PE, Ross R, Schwartz SM. An endothelial cell derived growth factor. *J Cell Biol* 1980; **85**: 467-72.

88. DiCorleto PE, Gadjusek CM, Schwartz SM, Ross R. Biochemical properties of the endothelium-derived growth factor: Comparison to other growth factors. *J Cell Physiol* 1983; **114**: 339-45.

89. DiCorleto PE, Bowen Pope DF. Cultured endothelial cells produce a platelet-derived growth factor-like protein. *Proc Nat'l Acad Sci USA* 1983; **80**: 1919.

90. Collins T, Ginsburg D, Boss JM, et al. Cultured human endothelial cells express platelet-derived growth factor B chain: cDNA cloning and structural analysis. *Nature* 1985; **316**: 748.

91. Collins T, Pober JS, Gimbrone MA, et al. Cultured human endothelial cells express platelet-derived growth factor A chain. *Am J Pathol* 1987; **126**: 7-11.

92. Barrett TB, Gadjusek CM, Schwartz SM, McDougall JK, Benditt EP. Expression of the *sis* gene by endothelial cells in culture and *in vivo*. *Proc Nat'l Acad Sci USA* 1984; **81**: 6772-4.

93. Nilsson J, Sjolund M, Palmberg L, Thyberg J, Heldin C-H. Arterial smooth muscle cells in primary culture produce a platelet-derived growth-factor like protein. *Proc Nat'l Acad Sci USA* 1985; **82**: 4418-22.

94. Morisaki N, Kanzaki T, Fujiyama Y, et al. Secretion of a new growth factor, smooth muscle cell derived growth factor, distinct from platelet derived growth factor by cultured rabbit aortic smooth muscle cells. *FEBS Lets* 1988; **230**: 186-90.

95. Leibovich SJ, Ross R. A macrophage-dependent factor that stimulates the proliferation of fibroblasts *in vitro*. *Am J Pathol* 1975; **84**: 501.

96. Shimokado K, Raines EW, Madtes DK, et al. A significant part of the macrophage-derived growth factor consists of at least two forms of PDGF. *Cell* 1985; **143**: 277-86.

97. Martinet Y, Bitterman PB, Mornex J-F, Grotendorst GR, Martin GR, Crystal RG. Activating human monocytes express c-sis proto-oncogene and release a mediator showing PDGF-like activity. *Nature* 1986; **319**: 158-60.

98. Baird A, Mormede P, Bohlen P. Immunoreactive fibroblast growth factor in cells of peritoneal exudate suggests its identity with macrophage derived growth factor. *Biochem: Biophys Res Commun* 1985; **126**: 358-64.

99. Madtes DK, Raines EW, Sakariasson KS, et al. Induction of transforming growth factor alpha in activating human alveolar macrophages. *Cell* 1988; **63**: 285-93.

100. Assoian RK, Komoriya A, Meyers CA, Miller DM, Sporn MB. Cellular transformation by co-ordinated action of three peptide growth factors from human platelets. *Nature* 1984; **309**: 804-6.

101. Roberts AB, Sporn MB. Transforming growth factor beta. In: *Advances in Cancer Research, Volume 51*. New York, London: Academic Press, 1988; 107-45.

102. Childs CB, Proper JA, Tucker RF, Moses HL. Serum contains a platelet-derived transforming growth factor. *Proc Nat'l Acad Sci, USA* 1982; **79**: 5312-60.

103. Barrett TB, Benditt EP. *sis* (PDGF-chain) gene transcript levels are elevated in human atherosclerotic lesions compared to normal artery. *Proc Nat'l Acad Sci USA* 1987; **84**: 1099.

104. Wilcox JN, Smith KM, Williams LT, Schwartz SM, Gordon D. Platelet derived growth factor mRNA detection in human atherosclerotic plaques by in situ hybridization. *J Clin Invest* 1988; **82**: 1134-43.

105. Benditt EP, Benditt JM. Evidence for a monoclonal origin of human atherosclerotic plaques. *Proc Nat'l Acad Sci USA* 1973; **70**: 1753-6.

106. Lyon MF. Gene action in the X-chromosome of the mouse (Mus musculus, L). *Nature* 1961; **190**: 372-3.

107. Linder D, Gartler SM. Glucose-6-phosphate dehydrogenase mosaicism: utilisation as a cell marker in the study of leiomyomas. *Science* 1965; **150**: 67-9.

108. Pearson TA, Wang A, Solez K, Heptinstall RH. Clonal characteristics of fibrous plaques and fatty streaks from human aortas. *Am J Pathol* 1975; **81**: 379-87.

109. Pearson TA, Dillman JM, Solez K, Heptinstall RH. Clonal characterisation in layers of human atherosclerotic plaques. *Am J Pathol* 1978; **73**: 93.

110. Pearson TA, Dillman JM, Solez K, Heptinstall RH. Clonal markers in the study of the origin and growth of human atherosclerotic lesions. *Circ Res* 1978; **43**: 10.

111. Thomas WA, Reiner JM, Florentin RA, Scott RF. Population dynamics of arterial cells during atherogenesis: VIII. Separation of the roles of injury and growth stimulation in early aortic atherogenesis in swine originating in pre-existing intimal smooth muscle cell masses. *Exp Mol Pathol* 1979; **31**: 124-44.

112. Thomas WA, Florentin RA, Reiner JM, Lee WM, Lee KT. Alterations in population dynamics of arterial smooth muscle cells during atherogenesis. IV. Evidence for a polyclonal origin of hypercholesterolaemic diet-induced atherosclerotic lesions in young swine. *Exp Mol Pathol* 1976; **24**: 244-60.

113. Zavala C, Herner G, Fialkow PJ. Evidence for selection in cultured diploid fibroblast strains. *Exp Cell Res* 1978; **177**: 137.

114. Lee KT, Thomas WA, Janakidevi K, Krons M, Reiner JM, Borg KY. Mosaicism in female hybrid hares heterozygous for glucose-6-phosphate dehydrogenase (G-6-PD). I. General properties of a hybrid hare model with special reference to atherogenesis. *Exp Mol Pathol* 1981; **34**: 191.

115. Thomas WA, Kim DN. Atherosclerosis as a hyperplastic and/or neoplastic process. *Lab Invest* 1983; **48**: 245-55.

116. Benditt EP. Implications of the monoclonal character of human atherosclerotic plaques. *Beit Pathol* 1976; **158**: 433-44.

117. Benditt EP. The artery wall and the environment. In: *Fifth Paavo Nurmi Symposium. Thrombosis and blood-vessel wall interactions in coronary heart disease. Acta Med Scand* 1980; (unpublished).

118. Benditt EP, Barrett T, McDougall JK. Viruses in the etiology of atherosclerosis. *Proc Nat'l Acad Sci USA* 1983; **80**: 6386.

119. Penn A, Garte SJ, Warren L, Nesta D, Mindich B. Transforming gene in human atherosclerotic plaque DNA *Proc Nat'l Acad Sci USA* 1986; **83**: 7951.

120. Fabricant CG, Fabricant J, Litrenta MM, Minick CR. Virus- induced atherosclerosis. *J Exp Med* 1978; **148**: 335-40.

121. Fabricant CG. The consequence of infection with a herpes virus. *Adv Vet Sci Comp Med* 1985; **30**: 39.

122. Smith EB. The influence of age and atherosclerosis on the chemistry of the aortic intima. I. The lipids. *J Ath Res* 1965; **5**: 224-40.

123. Smith EB. The relationship between plasma and tissue lipids in human atherosclerosis. *Adv Lipid Res* 1974; **12**: 1.

124. Bottcher CJF. Phospholipids of atherosclerotic lesions in the human aorta. In: Jones RJ, ed. *Evolution of the Atherosclerotic Plaque*. Chicago; University Press, 1964: 109-16.

125. Bottcher CJF, Woodford FP, Romeny-Wachter CTH, van Houte EB, van Gent CM. Fatty acid distribution in lipids of the aortic wall. *Lancet* 1960; **i**: 1378-83.

126. Geer JC, Malcolm GT. Cholesteryl ester fatty acid composition of human aorta fatty streaks and normal intima. *Exp Mol Pathol* 1964; **4**: 500-7.

127. Smith EB, Evans PH, Downham MD. Lipid in the aortic intima. The correlation of morphological and chemical characteristics. *J Ath Res* 1967; **7**: 171-86.

128. Newman HAI, Zilversmit DB. Quantitative aspects of cholesterol flux in rabbit atheromatous lesions. *J Biol Chem* 1962; **237**: 2078-84.

129. Watts HF. Pathogenesis of human coronary artery atherosclerosis. Demonstration of serum lipoproteins in the lesions and of localized intimal enzyme defects by histochemistry. *Circulation* 1961; **24**: 1066.

130. Watts HF. Role of lipoproteins in the formation of atherosclerotic lesions. In: Jones RJ, ed. *Evaluation of the Atherosclerotic Plaque*. Chicago: University Press, 1963: 117-32.

131. Woolf N, Pilkington TRE. The immunohistochemical demonstration of lipoproteins in vessel walls. *J Pathol Bacteriol* 1965; **91**: 459-63.

132. Walton KW, Williamson N. Histological and immunofluorescent studies in the evolution of the human atheromatous plaque. *J Ath Res* 1968; **8**: 599-624.

133. Smith EB, Slater RS. Relationship between low density lipoprotein in aortic intima and serum-lipid levels. *Lancet* 1972; i: 463-9.

134. Brown MS, Goldstein JL. Receptor-mediated control of cholesterol metabolism. *Science* 1976; **191**: 150-4.

135. Goldstein JL, Brown MS. The low density lipoprotein pathway and its relationship to atherosclerosis. *Ann Rev Biochem* 1977; **46**: 897-930.

136. Brown MS, Kovanen PT, Goldstein JL. Regulation of plasma cholesterol metabolism. *Science* 1981; **191**: 150-4.

137. Brown MS, Goldstein JL. How LDL receptors influence cholesterol and atherosclerosis. *Sci Am* 1984; **251**: 58-66.

138. Steinberg D, Parthasarathy S, Carew TE, Khoo JC, Witzum JL. Beyond cholesterol. Modifications of low-density lipoprotein that increase its atherogenicity. *N Engl J Med* 1989; **320**: 915-24.

139. Buja LM, Kipa T, Goldstein JL, Watanabe Y, Brown MS. Cellular pathology of progressive atherosclerosis in the WHHL rabbit. An animal model of familial hypercholesterolemia. *Arteriosclerosis* 1983; **3**: 87-101.

140. Goldstein JL, Ho YK, Basu SK, Brown MS. Binding site on macrophages that mediate uptake and degradation of acetylated low density lipoprotein producing massive cholesterol deposition. *Proc Nat'l Acad Sci USA* 1979; **76**: 333-7.

141. Brown MS, Goldstein JL. Lipoprotein metabolism in the macrophage: implications for cholesterol deposition in atherosclerosis. *Ann Rev Biochem* 1983; **52**: 223.

142. Fogelman AM, Schechter I, Seager J, Hokom M, Child JS, Edwards PA. Malondialdehyde alteration of low density lipoproteins leads to cholesteryl ester accumulation in human monocyte-macrophages. *Proc Nat'l Acad Sci USA* 1980; **77**: 2214.

143. Henrikson T, Mahoney EM, Steinberg D. Enhanced macrophage degradation of low density lipoprotein previously incubated with cultured endothelial cells: recognition by receptors for isolated low density lipoproteins. *Proc Nat'l Acad Sci* 1982; **78**: 6499-503.

144. Henrikson T, Mahoney EM, Steinberg D. Enhanced macrophage degradation of biologically modified low density lipoprotein. *Arteriosclerosis* 1983; **3**: 149-59.

145. Parthasarathy S, Young SG, Witztum JL, Pittman RC, Steinberg D. Probucol enhances oxidative modification of low density lipoprotein. *J Clin Invest* 1986; **77**: 641-4.

146. Quinn MT, Parthasarathy S, Steinberg D. Endothelial cell-derived chemotactic activity for mouse peritoneal macrophages and the effect of modified forms of low-density lipoprotein. *Proc Nat'l Acad Sci USA* 1985; **82**: 5949.

147. Quinn MT, Parthasarathy S, Steinberg D. Lysophosphatidylcholine: A chemotactic factor for human monocytes and its potential role in atherogenesis. *Proc Nat'l Acad Sci* 1988; **85**: 2805-9.

148. Quinn MT, Parthasarathy S, Fong LG, Steinberg D. Oxidatively modified low density lipoproteins: Potential role in recruitment and retention of monocyte/macrophage during atherogenesis. *Proc Nat'l Acad Sci* 1987; **84**: 2995-8.

149. Steinberg D. Metabolism of lipoproteins and their role in the pathogenesis of atherosclerosis. In: Stokes J III, Mancini M, eds. *Atherosclerosis Reviews, Volume 18*. New York: Raven Press, 1988.

150. Cathcart MK, Morel DW, Chisholm GM III. Monocytes and neutrophils oxidise low density lipoprotein making it cytotoxic. *J Leucocyte Biol* 1985; **38**: 341.

151. Henrikson T, Evensen SA, Carlander B. Injury to human endothelial cells in culture induced by low density lipoproteins. *Scand J Clin Lab Invest* 1979; **39**: 361.

152. Estebauer H, Zollner H, Schaur RJ. Hydroxyalkenals: cytotoxic products of lipid peroxidation. *ISI Atlas of Science: Biochemistry* 1988; **1**: 311-7.

153. Steinbrecher UP. Oxidation of human low density results in derivatization of lysine residues of apolipoprotein B by lipid peroxide decomposition products. *J Biol Chem* 1987; **262**: 3603-8.

154. Estebauer H, Quehenberger O, Jurgens G et al. Effect of peroxidative conditions on human plasma low-density lipoproteins. In: Nigam, ed. *Lipid Peroxidation and Cancer*. Berlin, Heidelberg, Springer-Verlag, 1988; 203-13.

155. Carew TE, Schwenke DC, Steinberg D. Antiatherogenic effect of probucol unrelated to its hypercholesterolaemic effect: evidence that antioxidants *in vivo* can selectively inhibit low density lipoprotein degradation in macrophage-rich fatty streaks and slow the progression of atherosclerosis in the Watanabe heritable hyperlipidemic rabbit. *Proc Nat'l Acad Sci* 1987; **84**: 7725-9.

156. Kita T, Nagaro Y, Yukode M, et al. Probucol prevents the progression of atherosclerosis in Watanabe heritable hyperlipidemic rabbit, an animal model for familial hypercholesterolaemia. *Proc Nat'l Sci USA* 1987; **84**: 5928.

157. Haberland ME, Fong D, Cheng L. Malondialdehyde-altered protein occurs in atheroma of Watanabe Heritable Hyperlipidemic Rabbits. *Science* 1988; **241**: 215-8.

158. Palinski W, Rosenfeld ME, Yla-Herttuala S, et al. Low density lipoprotein undergoes oxidative modification *in vivo*. *Proc Nat'l Acad Sci* 1989; **86**: 1372-6.

159. Bevilacqua MP, Pober JS, Majeau GR, Cotran RS, Gimbrone MA Jr. Interleukin 1 (IL-1) induces biosynthesis and cell surface expression of procoagulant activity in human vascular endothelial cells. *J Exp Med* 1984; **160**: 618.

160. Bevilacqua MP, Pober JS, Wheeler ME, Cotran RS, Gimbrone MA Jr. Interleukin-1 activation of vascular endothelium: Effects on procoagulant activity and leucocyte adhesion. *Am J Pathol* 1985; **121**: 394.

161. Pober JS. Cytokine-mediated activation of vascular endothelium: Physiology and pathology. *Am J Pathol* 1988; **133**: 426-33.

162. Munro JM, Cotran RS. The pathogenesis of atherosclerosis: atherogenesis and inflammation. *Lab Invest* 1988; **58**: 249-61.

163. Hartung H-P, Kladetsky RG, Melnik B, Hennerici M. Stimulation of the scavenger receptor on monocytes-macrophages evokes release of arachidonic acid metabolites and reduced oxygen species. *Lab Invest* 1986; **55**: 209-16.

164. Jonasson L, Holm J, Skalli O, Bondjers G, Hansson GK. Regional accumulations of T Cells, macrophages, and smooth muscle cells in the human atherosclerotic plaque. *Arteriosclerosis* 1986; **6**: 131.

165. Jonasson L, Holm J, Skalli O, Gabbiani G, Hansson GK. Expression of class II transplantation antigen on vascular smooth muscle cells in human atherosclerosis. *J Clin Invest* 1985; **76**: 125.

166. Hansson GK, Jonasson L, Holm J, Claesson-Welsh L. MHC antigen expression in the atherosclerotic plaque: Smooth muscle cells express HLA-DR, HLA-DQ and the invariant gamma chain. *Clin Exp Immunol* 1986; **64**: 261-8.

167. Hansson GK, Jonasson L, Holm J, Clowes MM, Clowes AW. Gamma interferon regulates smooth muscle proliferation and Ia expression in vivo and in vitro. *Circ Res* 1988; **63**: 712-9.

168. Emeson EE, Robertson AL. T lymphocytes in aortic and coronary intimas. Their potential role in atherogenesis. *Am J Pathol* 1988; **130**: 369-70.

169. Shaper AG. Coronary heart disease; risks and reasons. *Curr Med Lit (Lond)* 1988; 1-18.

170. Robertson WB. The International Atherosclerosis Project. *Pathol Microbiol* 1967; **30**: 810-6.

171. Woolf N. *The Pathology of Atherosclerosis*. London: Butterworths, 1982.

172. Cooper R, Stamler J, Dyer A, Garside D. The decline in mortality from coronary heart disease – USA, 1968-75. *J Chron Dis* 1978; **31**: 709-20.

173. Strong JP, Guzman MA. Decrease in

coronary atherosclerosis in New Orleans. *Lab Invest* 1980; **43**: 297-301.

174. Stamler J, Berkson DM, Lindberg HA. Risk factors: their role in the etiology and pathogenesis of the atherosclerotic disease. In: Wissler RS, Geer JC, eds. *The Pathogenesis of Atherosclerosis*. Baltimore: Williams and Wilkins, 1972: 41-119.

175. Robertson WB. Some factors influencing the development of atherosclerosis. A survey of Jamaica, West Indies. *J Ath Res* 1962; **2**: 79-87.

176. Strong JP, Eggen DA, Oalmann MC. The natural history, geographic pathology and epidemiology of atherosclerosis. In: Wissler RW, Geer JC, eds. *The Pathogenesis of Atherosclerosis*. Baltimore: Williams and Wilkins, 1972: 20-40.

177. McGill HC Jr. Atherosclerosis: Problems in pathogenesis. In: Paoletti R, Gotto AM, eds. *Atherosclerosis Reviews II*. New York: Raven Press, 1977: 27-65.

178. Stamler J. The coronary drug project – findings with regard to estrogen, dextrothyroxine, clofibrate and niacin. In: Manning GW, Haust MD, eds. *Atherosclerosis: Metabolic, Morphologic and Clinical Aspects*. New York: Plenum Press, 1978: 52-75.

179. Huttunen JK, Enholm C, Kekki M, Nikkila EA. Post-heparin plasma lipoprotein lipase and hepatic lipase in normal human subjects – relationship to age, sex and triglyceride metabolism. In: Manning GW, Haust MD, eds. *Atherosclerosis: Metabolic, Morphologic and Clinical Aspects*. New York: Plenum Press, 1977; 146-8.

180. Arntzenius AC, van Gent CM, van der Voort H, Stegerrhoek CI, Styblo K. Reduced high density lipoproteins in women aged 40-41 using oral contraceptives. *Lancet* 1978; ii: 1221-3.

181. Keys A, Kimura N, Kusukawa A, Bronte-Stewart B, Larsen N, Keys MA. Lessons in serum cholesterol studies in Japan, Hawaii and Los Angeles. *Ann Int Med* 1958; **48**: 83-94.

182. Marmot MG. Hypercholesterolemia: A public health problem. In: Stokes J III, Mancini M, eds. *Atherosclerosis Reviews, Volume 18*. New York: Raven Press, 1988: 95-131.

183. Shekelle RB, Shyrock AM, Oglesby P, et al. Diet serum cholesterol and death from coronary heart disease. The Western Electric Study. *N Engl J Med* 1981; **304**: 65-70.

184. Solberg LA, Hjerman I, Helgeland A, Holme I, Lerne PA, Strong JP. Association between risk factors and atherosclerotic lesions based on autopsy findings in the Oslo study: A preliminary report. In: Schettler G, Goto Y, Hata Y, Klose G, eds. *Atherosclerosis IV*. Berlin: Springer-Verlag, 1977: 98-102.

185. Gotto AM. Cholesterol and atherosclerosis. *Lipid Rev* 1987; 1: 1-6.

186. Brown MS, Goldstein JL. Familial hypercholesterolaemia: Defective binding of lipoproteins to cultured fibroblasts associated with impaired regulation of 3-hydroxy-3-methylglutaryl coenzyme A reductase activity. *Proc Nat'l Acad Sci USA* 1973; **71**: 788-92.

187. Brown MS, Goldstein JL. The LDL receptor concept: clinical and therapeutic implications. In: Stokes J III, Mancini M, eds. *Atherosclerosis Reviews, Vol 18* 1988. New York: Raven Press.

188. National Cholesterol Education Program Expert Panel on Detection, Evaluation and Treatment of High Blood Cholesterol in Adults. (Report of) *Arch Intern Med* 1988; **148**: 36-69.

189. Anitschkow N, Chalatow S. Über experimentelle Cholesterinsteatose und ihre Bedeutung für die Enstehung einiger pathologische Prozesse. *Centralblatt für Allgemeine Pathologie* 1913; **24**: 1.

190. Koletsky S. Obese, spontaneously hypertensive rats – a model for the study of atherosclerosis. *Exp Mol Pathol* 1973; **19**: 53-60.

191. Russell JC, Amy RM. Early atherosclerotic lesions in a susceptible rat model, the LA/N corpulent rat. *Atherosclerosis* 1986; **60**: 119-29.

192. Watanabe Y. Serial inbreeding of rabbits with hereditary hyperlipidemia (WHHL-rabbit). Incidence and development of atherosclerosis and xanthoma. *Atherosclerosis* 1980; **36**: 261-8.

193. Kita T, Brown MS, Watanabe Y, Goldstein JL. Deficiency of low density lipoprotein receptors of the WHHL rabbit, an animal model of familial hypercholesterolemia. *Proc Nat'l Acad Sci* 1981; **78**: 2268-72.

194. Kita T, Brown MS, Bilheimer DW, Goldstein JS. Delayed clearance of very low density and intermediate density lipoproteins with enhanced conversion to low density lipoproteins in WHHL rabbit. *Proc Nat'l Acad Sci* 1982; **79**: 5693-7.

195. LaVille A, Turner PR, Pittilo RM, et al. Hereditary hyperlipidaemia in the rabbit due to overproduction of lipoproteins. I. Biochemical studies. *Arteriosclerosis* 1987; **7**: 105-12.

196. Crawford T. *The Pathology of Ischaemic Heart Disease*. London: Butterworth, 1977: 32.

197. Doll R. Prospects for prevention. *Br Med J* 1983; **286**: 445-53.

198. Russell MA, West JR, Jarvis MJ. Intravenous nicotine simulation of passive smoke to estimated dosage to exposed non-smokers. *Br J Addict* 1985; **80**: 201-6.

199. Hammond EC. Smoking in relation to diseases other than cancer. Total death rates. In: Richardson RG, ed. *Proc Second World Conf on Smoking and Health* 1972; 24-34.

200. Doll R, Hill AB. Mortality in relation to smoking. Ten years' observations of British doctor. *Bri Med J* 1964; 1: 1399-410.

201. Dawber TR, Kannell WB, Stokes J, Kagan A, Gordon T. Some factors associated with the development of coronary heart disease. Six years follow-up experience in the Framingham study. *Am J Public Health* 1959; **49**: 1349-56.

202. Doyle JT, Dawber TR, Kannel WB, Kinch SH, Kahn HA. The relationship of cigarette smoking to coronary heart disease; the second report of the combined experience of the Albany, NY and Framingham, Mass. studies. *JAMA* 1964; **190**: 886-90.

203. Sackett DL, Epid MS, Gibson RW, Bross IDJ, Pickren JW. Relationship between aortic atherosclerosis and the use of cigarettes and alcohol. *N Engl J Med* 1968; **279**: 1413-20.

204. Gordon T, Kannel WB, McGee D, Daber TR. Death and coronary attacks in man after giving up cigarette smoking. A report from the Framingham study. *Lancet* 1974; ii: 1345-8.

205. Strong JP, Richards ML. Cigarette smoking and atherosclerosis in autopsied men. *Atherosclerosis* 1976; **23**: 451.

206. Wilens SL, Plair CM. Cigarette smoking and arteriosclerosis. *Science* 1962; **138**: 875-977.

207. Auerbach O, Hammond EC, Garfinkel L. Smoking in relation to atherosclerosis in the coronary arteries. *N Engl J Med* 1965; **273**: 775-9.

208. Strong JP, Richards ML, McGill HC Jr, Eggen DA, McMurry MD. On the association of cigarette smoking with coronary and aortic atherosclerosis. *J Ath Res* 1969; **10**: 303-17.

209. Tracy RE, Toca VT, Strong JP, Richards ML. Relationship of raised atherosclerotic lesions to fatty streaks in cigarette smokers. *Atherosclerosis* 1981; **38**: 347-57.

210. Asmussen I. Ultrastructure of the human placenta at term. Observations on placentas from newborn children of smoking and non-smoking mothers. *Acta Obstet Gynecol Scand* 1977; **65**: 119-26.

211. Asmussen I. Ultrastructure of human umbilical veins. Observations on veins from newborn children of smoking and non-smoking mothers. *Acta Obstet Gynecol Scand* 1978; **57**: 253-5.

212. Asmussen I. Arterial changes in infants of smoking mothers. *Postgrad Med J* 1978; **54**: 200-4.

213. Asmussen I. Chromatin changes of endothelial cells in umbilical arteries in smokers. *Clin Cardiol* 1982; **5**: 653-6.

214. Asmussen I. Ultrastructure of the umbilical arteries from newborn smoking and non-smoking mothers. *Acta Pathol Scand* 1982; **90**: 375.

215. Asmussen I. Ultrastructure of the umbilical artery from a newborn delivered at term by a mother who smoked 80 cigarettes per day. *Acta Pathol SCand* 1982; **90**: 397.

216. Asmussen I, Kjeldsen K. Intimal

ultrastructure of human umbilical arteries. Observations from arteries from newborn children of smoking and non-smoking mothers. *Circ Res* 1975; **36**: 579-89.

217. Bylock A, Bondjers G, Jannson I, Hansson HA. Surface ultrastructure of human arteries with special reference to the effects of smoking. *Acta Pathol Microbiol Scand (A)* 1979; **87**: 201-9.

218. Woolf N, Wilson-Holt N. Cigarette smoking and atherosclerosis. In: Greenhalgh RM, ed. *Smoking and Arterial Disease*. Bath: Pitman Medical, 1981: 46-59.

219. Bazin M, Turcotte H, Lagace R, Boutet M. Effets cardiovasculaires de la fumée de cigarette chez le rat. Etude de la perméabilité endotheliale et capillaire myocardique chez le rat. *Rev Can Biol* 1981; **40**: 263-76.

220. Sieffert GF, Keown K, Moore SW. Pathologic effect of tobacco smoke inhalation on arterial intima. *Surg Forum* 1981; **32**: 333.

221. Pittilo RM, Mackie IJ, Rowles PM, Machin SJ, Woolf N. Effects of cigarette smoking on the ultrastructure of rat thoracic aorta and its ability to produce prostacyclin. *Thromb Haemost* 1982; **48**: 173-6.

222. Bull HA, Pittilo RM, Blow CJ, et al. The effects on nicotine of PGI_2 production by rat endothelium. *Thromb Haemost* 1985; **54**: 472-4.

223. Booyse RM, Osikowicz G, Quarfoot AJ. Effects of chronic oral consumption of nicotine on the rabbit aortic endothelium. *Am J Pathol* 1981; **102**: 229-38.

224. Booyse RM, Osikowicz G, Radek J. Effect of nicotine on cultured bovine aortic endothelial cells. *Thromb Res* 1981; **23**: 169-85.

225. Nadler JL, Velasco JS, Horton R. Cigarette smoking inhibits prostacyclin production. *Lancet* 1983; **i**: 1248-50.

226. Reinders JH, Brinkman HJM, van Mourik JA, de Groot PG. Cigarette smoke impairs endothelial cell prostacyclin production. *Arteriosclerosis* 1986; **6**: 15-23.

227. Madsen H, Dyerberg J. Cigarette smoking and its effect on the platelet-vessel wall interaction. *Scand J Clin Lab Invest* 1984; **44**: 203-6.

228. Belch JJ, McArdle BM, Burns P, Lowe GDO, Forbes CD. The effects of acute smoking on platelet behaviour, fibrinolysis and haemorheology in habitual smokers. *Thromb Haemost* 1984;**51**: 6-8.

229. Hladovec J. Endothelial injury by nicotine and its prevention. *Experentia* 1978; **34**: 1585-6.

230. Prerovsky I, Hladovec J. Suppression of the desquamating effect of smoking on the human endothelium by hydroxyethylrutosides. *Blood Vessels* 1979; **16**: 239-40.

231. Davis JW, Shelton L, Eigenberg DA, Hignite CE, Watanabe IS. Effects of tobacco and non-tobacco cigarette smoking on

endothelium and platelets. *Clin Pharmacol Ther* 1985; **37**: 529-33.

232. Pittilo RM, Nicholson LJ, Clarke JMF, Blow CM, Woolf N. Cigarette smoke induced cytotoxicity of peritoneal mesothelial cells. *Br J Exp Pathol* 1985; **66**: 365-70.

233. Becker CG, Hajjar DP, Hefton JM. Tobacco constituents are mitogenic for arterial smooth muscle cells. *Am J Pathol* 1985; **120**: 1-5.

234. Meade TW, Imeson J, Stirling Y. Effects of changes in smoking and other characteristics on clotting factors and the risk of ischaemic heart disease. *Lancet* 1987; **ii**: 986-8.

235. Bierman EL. Diabetes mellitus, hyperlipidaemia and atherosclerosis. *Lipid Rev* 1989; **3**: 19-22.

236. Krolewski AS, Kolinsky EJ, Warram JH, et al. Magnitude and determinants of coronary artery disease of juvenile onset; insulin-dependent diabetes mellitus. *Am J Cardiol* 1987; **59**: 750-5.

237. Robertson WB, Strong JP. Atherosclerosis in persons with hypertension and diabetes mellitus. *Lab Invest* 1968; **18**: 538-51.

238. Rhoads GG, Blackwelder WE, Stemmerman GN, Hayashi T, Kagan A. Coronary risk factors and autopsy findings in Japanese-American men. *Lab Invest* 1978; **38**: 304-11.

239. Pyorala K, Savolainen E, Kaukola S, Haapakoski J. Plasma insulin as coronary heart disease factor: Relationship to other risk factors and predictive value during 9.5-year follow-up of the Helsinki Policeman Study population. *Acta Med Scand* 1985; **701 (Suppl)**: 38-52.

240. Rose AG. Review of primary prevention trials. *Am Heart J* 1987; **114**: 1013-7.

241. La Ville AE, Seddon AM, Shaikh M, Rowles PM, Woolf N, Lewis B. Primary prevention of atherosclerosis by lovastatin in a genetically hyperlipidaemic rabbit strain. *Atherosclerosis* 1989; **78**: 205-10.

242. Henry PD, Bentley KI. Suppression of atherogenesis in cholesterol fed rabbits treated with nifedipine. *J Clin Invest* 1981; **68**: 1366-9.

243. Ginsberg R, Davis K, Bristow MR, McKennett K, Kodsi SR, Billingham ME, Schroeder JS. Calcium antagonists suppress atherogenesis in aorta but not in the intramural coronary arteries of cholesterol-fed rabbits. *Lab Invest* 1983; **49**: 154.

244. Stender S, Stender I, Nordestgaard B, Kjeldsen K. No effect of nifedipine on atherosclerosis in cholesterol-fed rabbits. *Arteriosclerosis* 1984; **4**: 389.

245. Van Niekerk JLM, Hendriks Th, DeBoer HHM, Van't Laar A. Does nifedipine suppress atherogenesis in WHHL rabbits. *Atherosclerosis* 1984; **53**: 91.

246. Blumlein SL, Sievers R, Kidd P, Parmley WW. Mechanism of protection

from atherosclerosis by verapamil in the cholesterol-fed rabbit. *Am J Cardiol* 1984; **54**: 884-9.

247. Stein O, Lettersdorf E, Stein Y. Verapamil enhances receptor mediated endocytosis of low-density lipoproteins by aortic cells in culture. *Arteriosclerosis* 1985; **15**: 35-44.

248. Willis AJ, Nagel B, Churchill V, Whyte MA, Smith DL, Mahmud I, Puppione DL. Anti atherosclerotic effects of nicardipine and nifedipine in cholesterol-fed rabbits. *Arteriosclerosis* 1985; **5**: 250-5.

249. Ishikawa Y, Watanabe N, Okamoto R, Watanabe Y, Fukuzaki H. Nifedipine suppressed atherosclerosis in cholesterol-fed rabbits but not in Watanabe heritable hyperlipidemic rabbits. *Atherosclerosis* 1987; **64**: 79-80.

250. Handley DA, van Valen RG, Melden MK, Saunders RN. Suppression of rat carotid lesion development by the calcium channel blocker PN 200-110. *Am J Pathol* 1986; **124**: 88-93.

251. Lichtlen PR, Hugenholtz P, Rafflenbeul W, Jost S, Hecker H. Retardation of the progression of coronary artery disease with nifedipine. Results of INTACT. *Circulation* 1989; **80**.

252. Brozek J, Wells S, Keys A. Medical aspects of semi-starvation in Leningrad (siege 1941-2). *Am Rev Soviet Med* 1946; **4**: 70-86.

253. Vartiainen I, Kanerva K. Arteriosclerosis and wartime. *Ann Med Intern Fenn* 1947; **36**: 748-58.

254. Malmros H. The relation of nutrition to health. A statistical study of the effect of the wartime on arteriosclerosis, cardiosclerosis, tuberculosis and diabetes. *Acta Med Scand* 1950; **246**: 137-50.

255. Strom A, Jensen RA. Mortality from circulatory disease in Norway, 1940-1945. *Lancet* 1951; **i**: 120-9.

256. Aschoff L. *Lectures in Pathology*. New York: Hoeber, 1924; 131-53.

257. Beitzke H. Zür Entstehung der Atherosklerose. *Virchows Arch Pathol Anat* 1928; **267**: 625-47.

258. Armstrong ML. Connective tissue changes in regression. In: Schettler G, Goto Y, Hata Y, Klose G, eds. *Atherosclerosis IV*. Berlin: Springer Verlag, 1976; 405-13.

259. Bond MG, Bullock BC, Lehner WDM, Clarkson TB. Regression of atherosclerosis at plasma cholesterol levels achievable in man. In: Schettler G, Goto Y, Hata Y, Klose G, eds. *Atherosclerosis IV*. Berlin: Springer-Verlag, 1977: 278-80.

260. Daoud AS, Jarmolych J, Augustyn JM, et al. Regression in advanced atherosclerosis in swine. *Arch Path Lab Med* 1976; **100**: 372-9.

261. Wissler RW, Vesselinovitch D. Animal model of regression. In: Schettler G, Goto Y, Hata Y, Klose G, eds. *Atherosclerosis IV*. Berlin: Springer-Verlag, 1977: 377-85.

262. Malinow MR. Atherosclerosis:

Progression, regression, and resolution. *Am Heart J* 1984; **108**: 1523.

263. Higgins CB, Kaufmann L, Crooks LE. Magnetic resonance imaging of the cardiovascular system. *Am Heart J* 1985; **109**: 136-52.

264. Brown BG, Bolson E, Frimer M, Dodge HT. Quantitative coronary arteriography-estimation of dimensions, hemodynamic resistence and atheroma mass of coronary artery lesions during the arteriogram and digital computation. *Circulation* 1977; **55**: 329-37.

265. Arntzenius AC. Regression of atherosclerosis. *Horm Met Res* 1988; **19 (Suppl I)**: 19-22.

266. Blankenhorn DH. Angiographic evidence of atherosclerosis regression in man. In: Schettler G, Goto Y, Hata Y, Klose G, eds. *Atherosclerosis IV.* Berlin: Springer-Verlag, 1977: 414-21.

267. Blankenhorn DH, Brooks SH, Selzer RH, Barndt R Jr. The rate of atherosclerosis change during treatment of hyperlipoproteinemia. *Circulation* 1978; **57**: 355-61.

268. Lewis B. Progression and regression in atherosclerosis. *Lipid Rev* 1988; **2**: 33-8.

269. San Marco ME, Silvester RH, Brooks SH, Blankenhorn DH. Risk factor reduction and changes in coronary angiography. *Circulation* 1976; **54 (Suppl II)**: 140.

270. Duffield RGM, Lewis B, Miller NE, Jamieson CE, Brunt JNH, Colchester ACF. Treatment of hyperlipidaemia retards progression of symptomatic femoral atherosclerosis: A randomised controlled trial. *Lancet* 1983; 639-42.

271. Arntzenius AC, Kromhout D, Barth JD, et al. Diet, lipoproteins and progression of coronary atherosclerosis. *N Engl J Med* 1985; **312**: 805-11.

272. Brensike JF, Levy RI, Kelsey SF, et al. Effects of therapy with cholestyramine on progression of coronary arteriosclerosis: results of the NHLBI Type II coronary intervention study. *Circulation* 1984; **69**: 313-24.

273. Blankenhorn DH, Nessim SA, Johnson RL, San Marco ME, Azen SP, Cashin-Hemphill L. Beneficial effects of combined colestipol-niacin therapy on coronary atherosclerosis and coronary venous bypass grafts. *JAMA* 1987; **257**: 3233-40.

2

Morphology and Natural History of Atherosclerotic Lesions in the Human Artery Tree

Chapter 1 has established atherosclerosis as a disease affecting the intima of medium-sized and large arteries, ranging from the aorta to the coronary and cerebral vessels. The disease does not affect small arteries less than 2 to 3 mm in diameter. The salient features of the disease (see Box) have a considerable bearing on the manner in which significant obstruction to flow is produced in the arterial lumen.

> The lesions are focal and not diffuse, hence the term 'atherosclerotic plaque'.
>
> The intima is thickened by smooth muscle proliferation and production in excess of extracellular matrix proteins, in particular, collagen.
>
> The plaques contain lipid both within foam cells and as a mass of extracellular cholesterol.

This chapter is concerned with how these processes lead to clinical symptoms. The clinical course of patients with ischaemic heart disease shows two patterns; there is an apparently slowly progressive phase which leads to chronic obstruction to coronary blood flow, punctuated by acute episodes such as myocardial infarction or unstable angina. The latter are now established as being due to acute thrombotic episodes which are a complication of the basic atherosclerotic process. Even in patients whose clinical course with stable exertional angina suggests a slowly progressing disease, sequential coronary arteriography shows that high-grade stenoses often appear suddenly, rather than developing slowly. High-grade stenoses do not always develop at sites of previous low-grade stenoses (1,2).

The growth of plaques is episodic and unpredictable.

Types of coronary atherosclerotic plaque in man

The traditional technique used by pathologists – slitting an artery open along the longitudinal axis, flattening out the artery and viewing the inner surface – obscures some aspects of plaque morphology, but this method is so widely used that what it reveals must be given consideration. The lesion of importance, in that their number determines the progress of the disease, is the raised plaque. Each plaque is elevated above the surrounding surface and is oval-shaped with the long axis in the direction of flow. The surface of an uncomplicated plaque appears to be smooth and the endothelium intact. It must, however, be emphasized that the endothelium is a single layer of cells and its integrity cannot be determined with certainty by its macroscopic appearances alone. The apparent uniformity of raised plaques as seen by pathologists is misleading; there is considerable variation in structure from one plaque to another. This variation is best appreciated by considering the histological appearances of plaques when viewed as cross-sections of intact arteries.

Eccentric versus concentric
Transverse sections reveal that smaller plaques and therefore, by implication, those which are newer, do not occupy the entire luminal circumference of the vessel, and are situated eccentrically (Figure 2.1). As a result, there is opposite the plaque an arc of normal vessel wall with a normal media and intima. Larger plaques may occupy the entire luminal circumference of the vessel; these are termed 'concentric'.

If the transverse sections are prepared from an artery in which the lumen has been distended at systolic pressure, two features may be noted (see Box).

The lumen is circular in shape.

The outward bulge of the plaque is greater than or equal to its inward bulge.

The outward bulge is associated with, and due to, a marked atrophy of the media behind the plaque (Figure 2.2). The internal elastic lamina is often completely disrupted with the broken ends visible at the lateral margins of the plaque. The clinical implication of the outward bulge is that it is impossible to assess the size of a plaque solely from an angiogram which only outlines the residual lumen. Angiography shows the degree to which the lumen opposite the plaque is reduced in diameter in comparison to its proximal or distal segment, but does no more than this.

Figure 2.1
The different forms of coronary atherosclerotic plaques, as seen in transverse section.

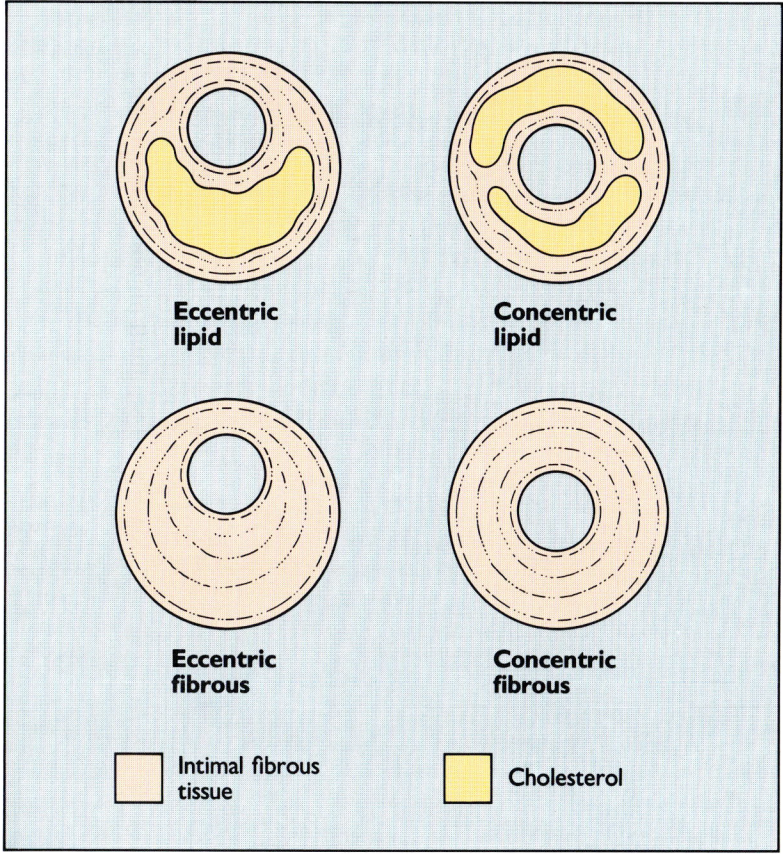

Eccentric lipid

Concentric lipid

Eccentric fibrous

Concentric fibrous

Intimal fibrous tissue

Cholesterol

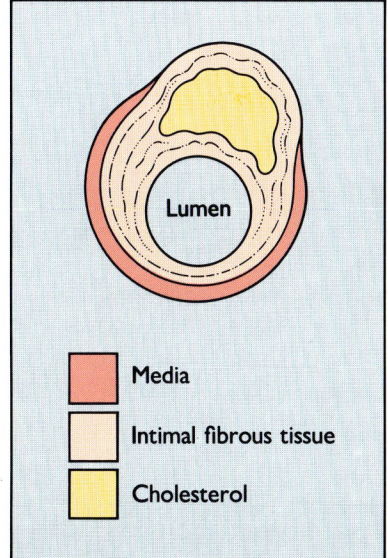

Lumen

Media

Intimal fibrous tissue

Cholesterol

Figure 2.2
A coronary plaque which bulges outward through the media. Part of the plaque lies outside of the original outline of the vessel wall.

Large plaques do not necessarily cause high-grade stenosis.

In arteries which have been fixed by distention at systolic pressure in the absence of medial tone (at *post mortem*), the lumen is round except when thrombus or calcified nodules project into the lumen. This does not indicate that the coronary artery lumen is round *in vivo*. Plaques are more rigid than the surrounding tissue and do not bend easily. When a rigid plaque is eccentric, tone in the normal vessel wall may produce an oval-shaped lumen. The crescentic or slit-like lumina so often illustrated in pathology texts and seen at angioscopy are, however, usually an artefact of low intraluminal pressure.

The reasons for the medial atrophy behind plaques is still not clear. It may be either a form of pressure atrophy or a hypoxic phenomenon due to the intimal thickening causing an increase in the distance of the medial smooth muscle cells from oxygenated blood in the lumen of the artery. The media of normal coronary arteries in man is avascular and not entered by vessels from the adventitia. Behind established plaques, however, new vessels enter the media from the adventitia and may extend as far as the intima at the base of the plaque itself. Such neovascularization may enhance access to the media of inflammatory cells, including monocytes which, when activated to release cytotoxins, may be another factor in causing a loss of medial smooth muscle cells.

The development of a plexus of vessels in the adventitia adjacent to a plaque, and the extensive neovascularization of the plaque itself, may be sufficiently pronounced so as to be visible as a blush on the external surface of the coronary arteries at surgery or autopsy (Figure 2.3). The adventitial plexus fills very readily on angiography (3) both in life and at autopsy and, when present in association with high-grade stenosis, may be responsible for some local collateral flow, although the small calibre of the adventitial vessels makes it unlikely that they are of functional significance.

Figure 2.3
Telangectasia over an atheromatous plaque in the right coronary artery. The increased adventitial vascularity is seen as a red blush on the visceral pericardium over the artery.

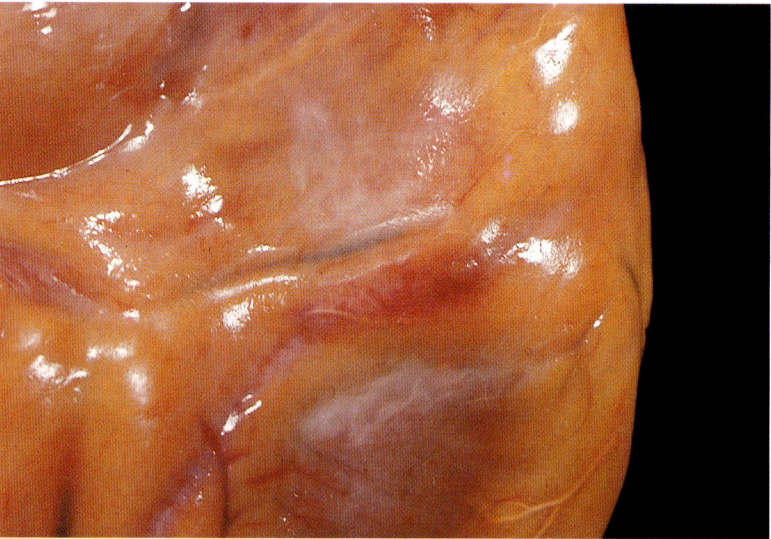

A proportion of patients with coronary atheroma show a florid infiltration of lymphocytes, plasma cells and monocytes in the adventitia adjacent to some or all of their plaques. These inflammatory cell infiltrates are restricted to the immediate vicinity of the plaque. The likely initiating factor is oxidized lipoprotein released from within the plaque, and there may be an element of 'autoimmunity' involved with the formation of antibodies to lipoproteins (4). The resulting local inflammatory response may be responsible for further destruction of the media and may also be an important mechanism in the formation of aneurysms in atherosclerotic aortas.

Fibrous versus lipid-rich plaques

As there is considerable variation in the constituents of the raised plaque in coronary arteries, a 'standard' plaque does not exist. At one end of the spectrum are solid plaques which are composed almost entirely of collagen containing a variable number of smooth muscle cells; lipid is virtually absent. At the other end of the spectrum are plaques which are rich in lipid and contain a pool of extracellular cholesterol (5). Between these extremes are plaques containing a collagenous matrix interspersed with lipid-filled foam cells. Usually, a variety of plaque types within this spectrum is present but, in some cases, the plaque population is relatively homogeneous. The pathogenesis of the different types of raised plaque and whether there is a developmental sequence in man is not known. As yet, there is no method available of typing plaques in man *in vivo* to follow their natural history.

The lipid-rich plaque, which contains a pool of extracellular cholesterol, is important because it is responsible for most episodes of major coronary thrombosis (6,7). In arteries which have been distended by pressure during laboratory prepara-

Figure 2.4

Histology (transverse section) of an eccentric lipid-rich coronary plaque containing a crescent-shaped pale-staining area (from which lipid has been dissolved during tissue processing). The lipid pool is separated from the lumen of the artery (L) by the plaque cap comprising connective tissue and smooth muscle cells. Endothelial cells are not seen at this low magnification.

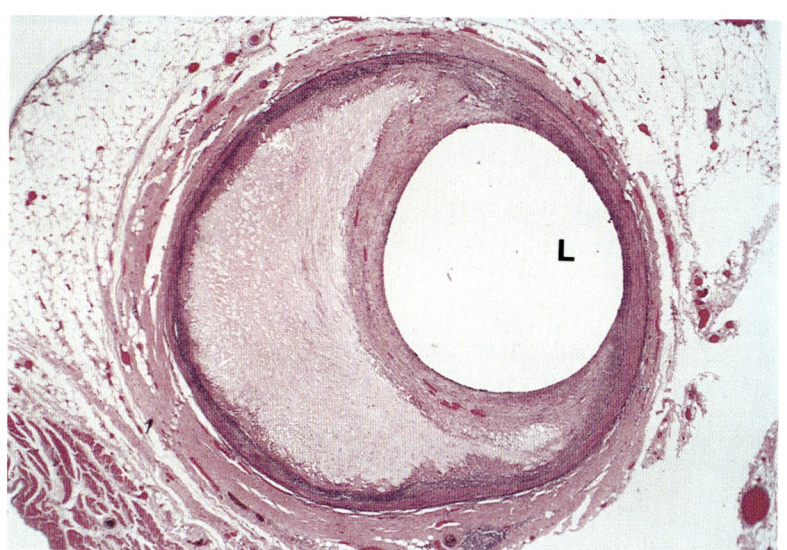

tion, the lipid pool shows as a crescent-shaped space, filled with cholesterol crystals and esters, within the connective tissue matrix of the intima (Figure 2.4). At surgery or autopsy, this lipid can be seen, and felt, to have the consistency of toothpaste. The lipid pool is separated from the arterial lumen by a cap of fibrous tissue containing smooth muscle cells. The margins of the pool are surrounded by lipid-filled foam cells, which have been demonstrated to be predominantly of monocyte/macrophage origin (8).

Plaque calcification

Plaques may or may not develop calcification. When it develops, it occurs deep within the intima close to the base of the plaque adjacent to the media and is characteristically seen as a thin shell or plate of calcium within the fibrous tissue. This form of calcification may develop in both fibrous and lipid-rich plaques. A different pattern, involving the formation of nodular masses of calcium within the intima, is seen in individuals over 70 years of age. As calcification occurs deep within the intima, it does not directly contribute to stenosis of the lumen. Calcification which is visible on radiography, particularly in younger individuals, indicates the presence of extensive atheroma and, thus, a high likelihood of stenosis, but there is no direct relationship between calcification and stenosis.

Endothelium overlying plaques in man

Normal arteries are lined with a single layer of endothelial cells which cover the intimal surface. In normal vessels, these endothelial cells are arranged with their long axes in the direction of blood flow. Denudation injury, the removal of only the endothelial cells in a focal area, exposes the subendothelial connective tissue to platelets, leading to the formation of a small microthrombus. Numerous experimental models of minor single episodes of denudation injury in normal arteries (see Chapter 1) have shown that the thrombus, a single layer of platelets, usually does not grow, and endothelial continuity may be rapidly restored. There is, however, some variation between species in the speed with which endothelial continuity is restored.

Figure 2.5
Scanning electron micrograph of an intact endothelial surface over a plaque in man. The endothelial cells have lost their alignment in the direction of flow, but there is no denudation.

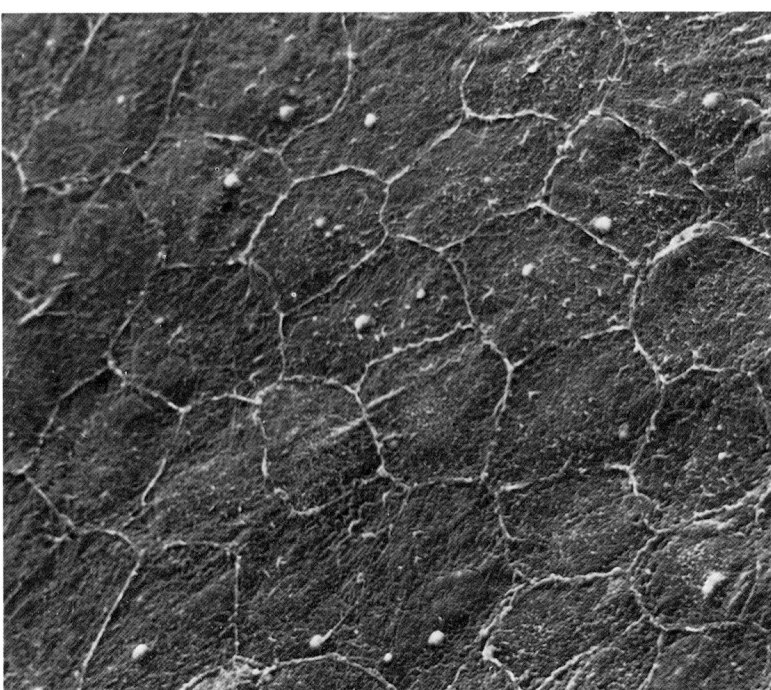

In experimental animals in which atherosclerosis has been induced by high-lipid diets, it has been firmly established that there is focal endothelial denudation over many raised plaques, particularly in association with infiltration of the superficial layers of the intima by lipid-laden macrophages (9).

Studies involving examination of human atherosclerotic coronary arteries obtained at cardiac transplantation have confirmed that focal endothelial denudation occurs over some raised plaques (10). The endothelium over plaques even when intact has lost the normal orientation of cells in the direction of flow (Figure 2.5). The small size of these denudation lesions and their resulting thrombi must be emphasized. These areas represent a loss of less than 20 endothelial cells, and the thrombi consist of a single layer of platelets (Figure 2.6). These microthrombi can be detected only by scanning electron microscopy, and are not detectable by any form of angiography.

The presence of focal denudation injury in atherosclerotic arteries in man may be the ultimate morphological expression of a more widespread functional abnormality of what must be a constantly regenerating endothelial surface.

Figure 2.6
Scanning electron micrograph of focal endothelial denudation injury. An endothelial cell has been lost and the exposed subendothelial tissue is covered by a layer of platelets and a few fibrin strands.

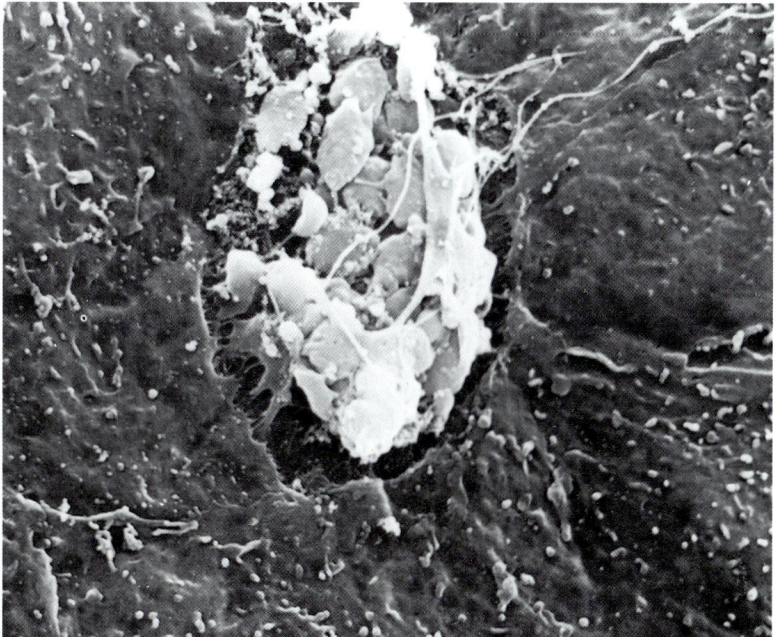

Initiation of thrombosis in atheroma

Microthrombi arising as a result of focal denudation of endothelium are an integral part of the atheromatous process once raised plaques have formed, but the clinical course of patients with coronary atherosclerosis is often punctuated by more major thrombi that significantly interfere with blood flow. Major intraluminal thrombi can be detected both by post-mortem and in-vivo angiography.

With very rare exceptions, major thrombi are not found in normal coronary arteries; they are the result of events which occur in, or over, an atheromatous plaque. Reconstruction of the microanatomy of the intima underlying these thrombi post mortem provides considerable insight into the mechanisms by which a previously stable plaque becomes an unstable plaque with an intensely thrombogenic surface.

Morphological studies show that approximately 75% of major thrombi are initiated by tearing of the plaque, which exposes large amounts of collagen and lipid to the blood. This tearing process has also been referred to as fissuring, cracking or rupture of the plaque and produces an 'injury' which extends deep into the intima. The remaining 25% of coronary thrombi are due to more superficial intimal injury in which endothelial loss alone is the predominant factor initiating thrombosis. The two processes, superficial and deep intimal injury (11), contrast each other in many respects (Figure 2.7).

Deep intimal injury

In deep intimal injury, the initiating event is a tear which extends from the lumen into the plaque itself. The form of plaque which most frequently undergoes this process has a lipid-rich core, and the tear extends from the lumen through the cap and into the lipid pool. The tears range from cracks or fissures measuring a hundred microns across to complete loss of the entire cap over several millimeters; the more major forms of plaque disruption are often termed 'plaque rupture' or 'ulceration'. Since the plaque cap is covered by an endothelial surface, concomitant endothelial denudation over a large area must also occur.

An episode of plaque fissuring is followed by a sequence of events with several possible end-points (Figure 2.8). All fissures allow blood from the lumen to enter the lipid pool. Within the lipid pool, platelets are exposed to collagen, crystalline cholesterol and oxidized low-density lipoprotein (LDL), leading to the formation of a platelet-rich thrombus within the plaque itself. Intraintimal thrombus considerably expands the plaque volume and radically alters its configuration. The platelet-preponderate structure of the thrombus within the plaque indicates that blood has entered and left the pool over a considerable period of time to allow sufficient accrual of

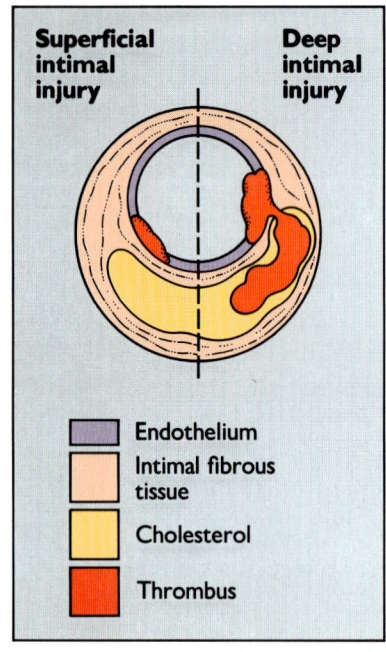

Superficial intimal injury | **Deep intimal injury**

Endothelium
Intimal fibrous tissue
Cholesterol
Thrombus

Figure 2.7
A comparison of the features of superficial and deep intimal injury. The most important distinction is the presence of intraintimal thrombosis in deep injury, which is absent in superficial injury.

Figure 2.8
Potential results of an episode of plaque fissuring.

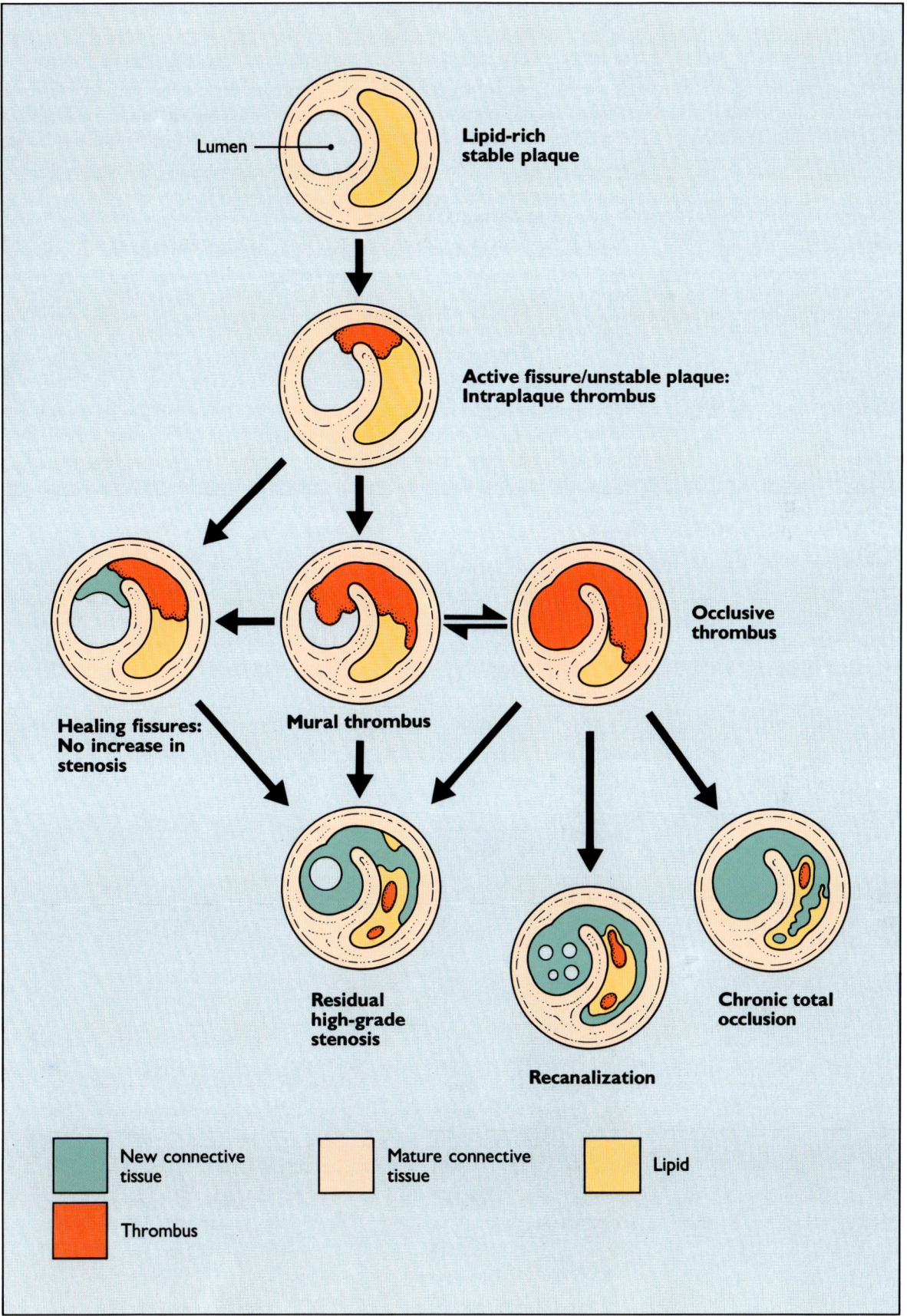

platelets. The structure of the thrombus is different from that which occurs in static blood.

Intimal injury of this magnitude inevitably invokes smooth muscle proliferation at the site and fissures often reseal. The likely sequence of events is that the fissure itself is blocked by a more fibrin-rich thrombus, which is rapidly invaded by smooth muscle cells which form collagen. On histology, the more mature collagen of the original plaque cap is retained as an outline, allowing recognition of recently 'healed' episodes of fissuring. Incarcerated thrombus remains within the plaque and slowly undergoes replacement by connective tissue. It may be that, in some instances, the lipid pool is totally obliterated, ultimately resulting in a fibrous plaque.

The process of plaque fissuring must, therefore, be seen as a mechanism for episodic plaque growth which may significantly increase the degree of stenosis over a very short period of time. This form of plaque growth does not involve the formation of thrombus within the lumen itself, and is responsible for the rapid progression of stenoses which may occur without associated acute clinical symptoms.

Post-mortem analysis of the coronary arteries of control subjects (those individuals who have a clearly identified cause of death other than ischaemic heart disease) confirms that a minor episode of recent plaque fissuring is common with raised plaques in the coronary arteries: 8% of control subjects without risk factors for ischaemic heart disease had such a lesion while, in subjects with hypertension, diabetes or previous myocardial infarction, the proportion rose to 16% (12). The latter figure probably indicates that this group has more raised plaques and, therefore, a greater risk of fissuring. In the con-

Figure 2.9
Histology showing a small intramyocardial artery, distal to a fissured plaque with mural thrombus, plugged by a mass of platelets. The platelets appear as purple dots.

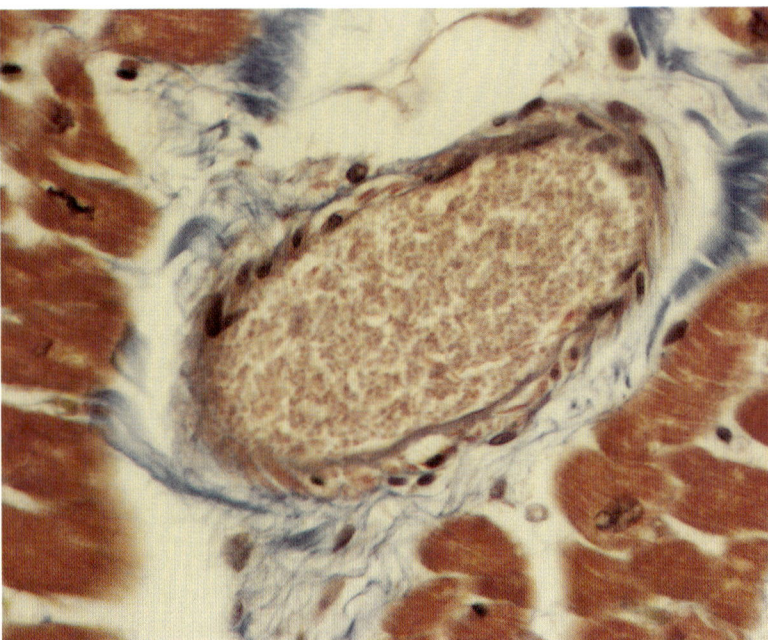

trol groups, the fissures themselves and the resulting intraintimal thrombi are smaller than those found in association with clinically expressed ischaemic heart disease.

Thus, it is clear that the majority of plaque fissures reseal and heal, producing a higher degree of stenosis with each episode. A minority of episodes, however, progress to the formation of an intraluminal thrombus.

> An episode of plaque fissuring is a stimulus to the formation of intraluminal thrombosis, but is not inevitably followed by intraluminal thrombosis.

Intraluminal thrombus initially forms within and over the fissure itself, and is composed of densely packed fibrin which is covered by a layer of platelets. A pedunculated mass of thrombus (mural thrombus) often projects into the lumen. At this stage, distal embolization may occur and the microemboli consist predominantly of platelet masses derived from the surface layer of the mural thrombus (Figure 2.9).

A further proportion of plaque fissures progress *via* mural thrombus to become occlusive thrombus. The intraluminal thrombus at this third and final stage of thrombosis comprises a network of fibrin in which numerous red cells are enmeshed; the platelet component is small (Figure 2.10). This thrombus extends proximally and distally from the plaque which has undergone fissuring usually as far as the entry of a major branch. Distal propagation may extend throughout the whole artery, particularly the right coronary artery.

Figure 2.10
Reconstruction of a plaque fissure with occluding thrombus showing the different structure of each stage in the process. The initial intraplaque thrombus is platelet-rich; the thrombus within the fissure and projecting into the lumen is fibrin-rich. The final occluding thrombus is a loose network of fibrin packed with red cells.

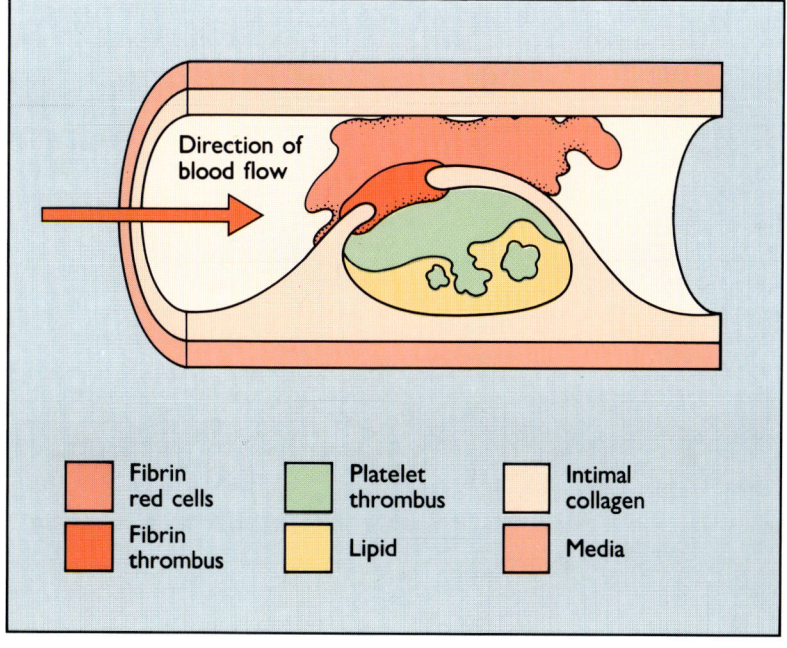

Direction of blood flow

Fibrin red cells	Platelet thrombus	Intimal collagen
Fibrin thrombus	Lipid	Media

Resolution of coronary thrombosis
Sequential angiograms in living patients who have had a sudden occlusion of a coronary artery show that a proportion of the vessels spontaneously reopen, and the use of fibrinolytic therapy very considerably increases this proportion. Pathological studies of the arteries of large numbers of patients who have died of acute regional infarction show the various patterns (see Boxes) that can evolve, following an episode of occlusive thrombosis (see Figure 2.8).

Possible arterial patterns of response to occlusive thrombosis

Antegrade flow is restored by lysis of the third and final stage of intraluminal thrombus. The degree of residual stenosis depends on the size of the original plaque, the degree of plaque expansion due to the intraintimal thrombus at the time of fissuring, and the degree of connective tissue proliferation in the repair phase.

Antegrade flow is restored by recanalization of the occlusive thrombus by small vessels that enter during the healing phase. The most common pattern is one of numerous smaller vessels within the original lumen (Figure 2.11) but, on occasion, there are as few as two new channels. While antegrade flow can be shown through the multichanneled lumina both by in-vivo and post-mortem angiography, the functional importance of such flow is not known.

The thrombus is eventually replaced by fibrous tissue rather than being removed by lysis, and a chronic total occlusion results.

Factors influencing the various possible consequences of plaque-fissuring

The size of the lipid pool: To allow the development of a large intraintimal thrombus, a large space must be available. Plaques in which the fibrous cap is relatively thin and covers a large pool are able to expand rapidly and bulge into the lumen.

The degree of pre-existing stenosis: High-grade stenosis may favour low flow, thus encouraging thrombus formation.

The relative size of the intraluminal and intraintimal thrombus: Some plaque fissures result in a large intraintimal thrombus. Such expanded plaques alone may totally obstruct the lumen without need for an accompanying large intraluminal component. Other fissures have a minor intraplaque component and a major intraluminal component. The reasons for the exaggerated thrombotic potential in the face of a small intimal injury may lie in the thrombotic/lytic potential of the patient at that time.

The size of the defect in the plaque cap: Major tears at the extreme end of the spectrum may allow extrusion of plaque contents into the lumen. In some cases, the lumen is occluded by a plug of thrombus containing cholesterol and fragments of the cap itself mixed with thrombus. These thrombi are inherently less likely to be removed by spontaneous lysis and lead to chronic complete obstruction.

Figure 2.11
Recanalized artery seen (left) on angiography and (right) on histology (transverse section). New vascular channels have formed within the original lumen.

Superficial intimal injury

A minor, but still significant, proportion of major coronary thrombi are not related to deep intimal injury with plaque fissuring, but are superimposed on what appears to be an intact

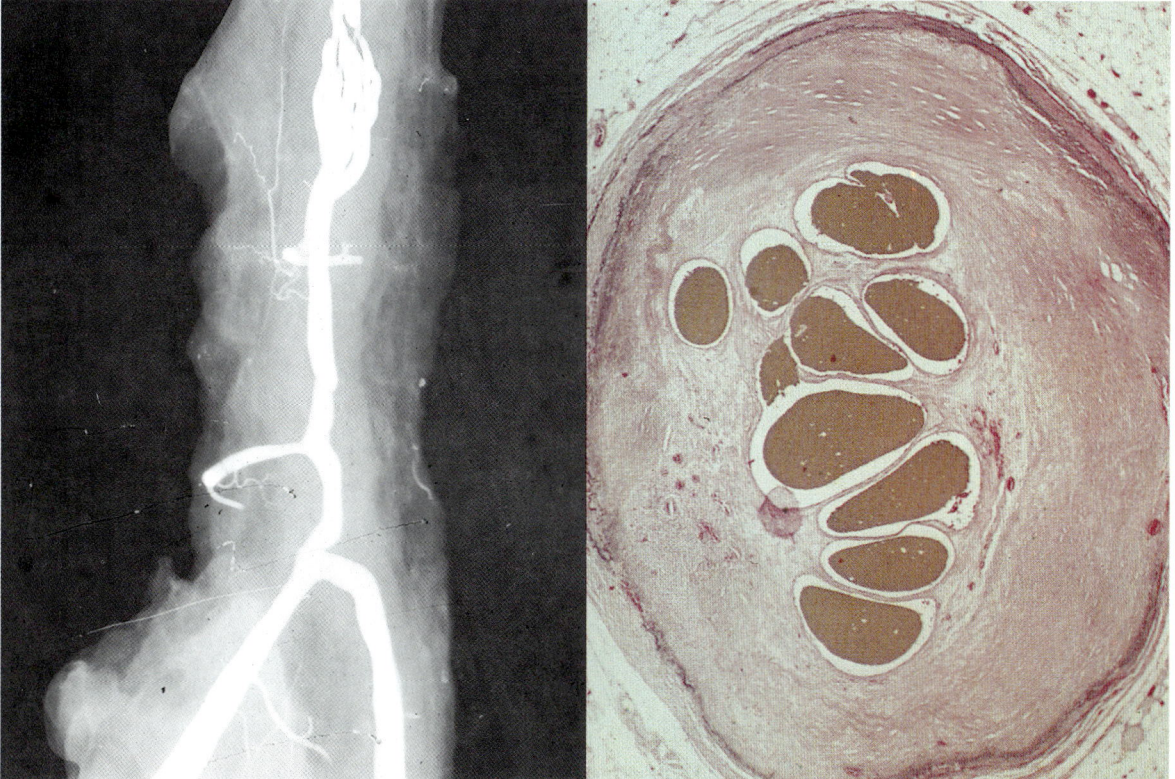

Figure 2.12
Two mural thrombi projecting into the lumen of a coronary artery. The thrombi are applied to the surface of an otherwise intact plaque with no evidence of deep fissuring.

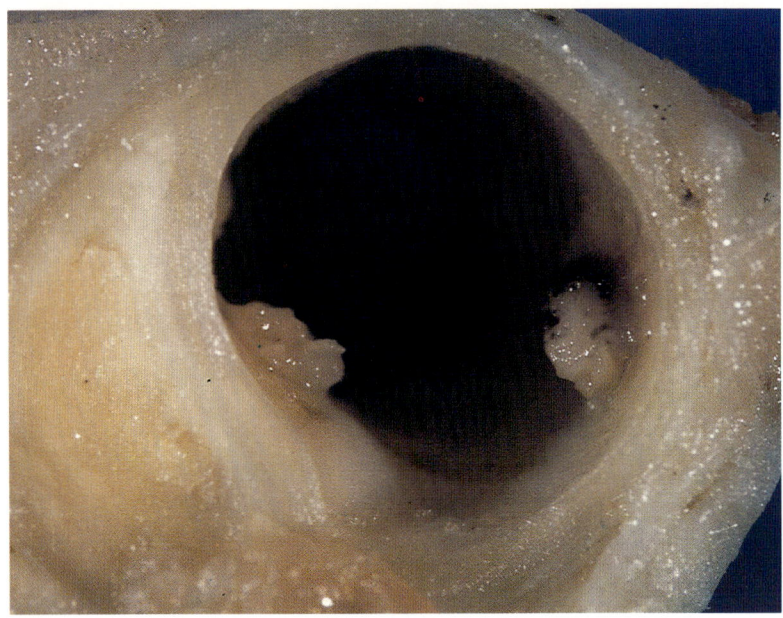

plaque (Figure 2.12). The features of these thrombi differ from those which result from deep injury (see Box).

> There is a greater association with previous high-grade stenosis.
>
> There is an association with macrophage infiltration in the form of lipid-filled foam cells in the superficial layers of the intima. Endothelial loss is apparent in these areas.
>
> These lesions are more common in smaller arteries such as the left marginal branch.

The process appears to represent a severe and widespread endothelial loss and can be considered to be the ultimate development of the microthrombi that develop over otherwise stable plaques.

Superficial endothelial denudation may follow flow- and shear-stress alterations distal to high-grade stenoses as evidenced by experimental studies (13) or it may be associated, as in experimental animals, with accumulation of macrophages immediately beneath the endothelial surface (14).

Pathogenesis of plaque fissuring and intimal tearing

Tearing of any connective tissue structure may result from either the tissue being exposed to an increased load or being weakened in its ability to resist a mechanical force. Analysis of spontaneous intimal tears leading to coronary thrombosis in man (7) shows that the great majority occur in plaques which have a lipid pool occupying an arc of the intima and in which the pool is not buttressed internally by collagen to support the plaque cap. Most tears occur at the lateral margin of the plaque where the cap joins the more normal intima.

The arterial wall is subject to considerable circumferential tensile stress on each systolic pulse. Any structure within the intima, such as a soft mass of lipid unable to carry a load, raises the wall stress elsewhere. When the soft mass is eccentrically positioned, there is a focus of stress on the cap at exactly the site where most spontaneous tears occur (7).

Analysis of plaque caps in the aorta, comparing ruptured and non-ruptured plaques, shows the former to have higher concentrations of lipid-filled macrophages; on mechanical testing, caps which have an open lattice of collagen infilled with lipid-laden foam cells are not as strong as caps made up of uniformly dense collagen. The weakness of a collagenous structure which is infiltrated by foam cells is well illustrated by rupture of the Achilles tendon in patients with xanthomatosis.

Coronary arteries in patients with angina

The clinical symptoms of angina extend across a spectrum from patients whose pain is consistently related to a predictable level of exercise (stable exertional angina) or to an increase in myocardial oxygen demand due to rises in heart rate and blood pressure, through to those patients who have angina at rest and whose symptoms increase in magnitude over several days (unstable angina). Between these extremes are patients whose stable angina is complicated by transient myocardial ischaemia at rest, sometimes with pain, but often without (silent ischaemia). It is accepted that the term 'unstable angina' implies that acute myocardial infarction has not occurred, although there is a risk that it will in the near future. It is unlikely that any single pathogenetic mechanism can cover such a broad spectrum of angina; it is now established that chronic stable angina is associated with fixed high-grade stenosis, unstable angina with thrombosis but without total occlusion and, in both, a contribution is made by alterations in vasomotor tone either at the site of the lesions in the main coronary arteries or in the distal vascular bed. Many patients probably have a combination of all these mechanisms at some time in the course of their disease.

Coronary artery lesions in chronic stable angina

Angiographic studies in life and *post mortem* confirm that stable angina that is directly related to an increase in myocardial oxygen demand is associated with discrete areas of high-grade stenosis in one or more of the major coronary arteries. High-grade stenosis is defined as lesions which cause narrowing of the lumen by more than 50% in diameter (equivalent to a 75% reduction in the cross-sectional area of the lumen). This definition is based on the fact that this degree of reduction in cross-sectional luminal area is required to significantly influence flow at any given pressure within a tube, and has been confirmed by clinical experience. However, the definition is, at best, crude.

The length of the stenotic segment also influences flow, probably by inducing turbulence (15,16). Serial stenoses reduce flow disproportionately to the degree of narrowing of each. Measurement of the degree of stenosis is difficult using either angiograms or histology. The former make the assumption that there is an adjacent reference segment of artery with a normal-sized lumen. However, the reference segment itself may have diffuse unrecognized atheroma and an already reduced cross-sectional lumen, thus leading to an underestimate of the degree of stenosis in the test segment. On histological examination, the area of the lumen is compared to that of the whole vessel at that point. Atherosclerotic arteries, however, have a considerably increase in their external diameter when compared to normal vessels, and the degree of stenosis at a given point may then be overestimated. Given these difficulties, it is not surprising that the absolute cross-sectional area of the lumen at any point is the ideal measurement to make (17), although crude assessment of stenoses based on visual assessment of arterial diameter from the angiogram has stood the test of clinical relevance, and is likely to continue in most centres.

Morphology of high-grade stenoses in stable angina
Detailed studies at post-mortem examination have been carried out on the morphology of high-grade lesions in patients with stable angina (18,19). The majority of these patients have been shown to have at least one arterial lesion which is the ultimate result of a previous occluding thrombus. The lesions are either chronic total obstructions and/or arterial segments containing a new multichanneled lumen (Figure 2.11). In an autopsy study of 54 patients with stable angina (19), 43 (78%) patients had such a recanalized segment. Of the 16 patients who had not had a previous myocardial infarction, 63% had such lesions also, demonstrating that total coronary artery occlusion is not inevitably followed by infarction.

When stenoses that were not the result of previous thrombotic occlusion were considered, there was an average of 8.3 segments with a more than 75% cross-sectional area of stenosis per patient. When patients without previous infarction were considered, this figure fell to 5.6 segments per case. The extent, severity and distribution of stenosis in any pathological series are biased in favour of those cases with triple-vessel disease and left main stem involvement. The results of clinical series based on angiography in living patients are more optimistic, showing a higher proportion with single-vessel disease.

The morphology of high-grade stenotic lesions in stable angina is of importance with regard to the potential for angioplasty and the possibility of vasomotor tone causing variations in the degree of stenosis at the site. Plaques may either be solid and fibrous or contain a pool of extracellular lipid; they may also be either concentric or eccentric. In the latter case, there is an arc of normal vessel wall opposite the plaque itself. Areas of high-grade stenosis can therefore be categorized as concentric fibrous, eccentric fibrous, eccentric lipid-rich or concentric lipid-rich (see Figure 2.1).

When a large number of high-grade stenotic lesions from a pool of patients with ischaemic heart disease are studied *post mortem*, the proportion of individual lesions reported to be eccentric, rather than concentric, ranges from 24% to over 70% (19-21). Group data, however, conceal a very wide range of individual variation. Some patients have no eccentric high-grade lesions while other patients have high-grade lesions which are all eccentric. It is probably more useful to consider that between 50 and 60% of patients with stable angina have one or more eccentric lesions (19).

It is now accepted that the degree of obstruction to flow can vary at the site of eccentric stenoses. It has been shown that the cross-sectional area of the lumen at points of eccentric stenosis can be increased or decreased pharmacologically (22). Abnormal vasomotor tonal responses appear to be a very reasonable explanation for transient ischaemia at rest in a patient whose main complaint is stable exertional angina. However, so far, there has been no formal proof that this is the mechanism, although eccentric lesions are more commonly found in patients with, rather than without, silent resting ischaemic attacks (23).

There is a similar wide variation in plaque types in the presence or absence of a pool of extracellular lipid as that for concentric or eccentric lesions. Some patients have no lipid-rich plaques while others have only this type of plaque, but most patients have a mixture of the two. There is, as yet, no angiographic criteria to distinguish coronary lipid-rich from fibrous plaques *in vivo*, although there are criteria which have been established in the aorta using magnetic resonance imaging (24).

Coronary artery lesions in unstable angina

The twin themes of thrombosis and arterial spasm are regarded as the mechanism for the episodes of resting ischaemia which characterize unstable angina and, in any given patient, it may be difficult to ascertain which mechanism is predominant. In general, the crescendo type of unstable angina, with rapid onset and acceleration of symptoms which either resolve rapidly or lead to acute infarction, is likely to be of thrombotic origin.

In-vivo angiographic studies comparing the morphology of the stenoses found in stable and unstable angina have consistently shown that there is no difference in the degree and extent of arterial narrowing (25). Stable angina is associated with both concentric and eccentric segments of narrowing which are smooth in outline (Type I; Figure 2.13). In contrast, most patients with unstable angina have one or more lesions which are eccentric and have a ragged or overhanging outline (Type II; Figure 2.14). Associated with a significant proportion of Type II lesions is the angiographic demonstration of intraluminal filling defect (26-28). These defects represent mural thrombus projecting into the coronary lumen, as has been confirmed at angioscopy (29). Angiography *in vivo* in comparison to angioscopy (29) is an ineffectual method of detecting thrombi, and all Type II stenoses probably have an element of intraluminal thrombosis.

Numerous pathological studies (30-32) have shown that a Type II angiographic morphology is indicative of a plaque which is undergoing fissuring and has reached the stage in which thrombus projects into the lumen, but antegrade flow is still present (Figure 2.15). It has therefore been established that, in a high proportion of patients with unstable angina, there is a 'culprit' lesion, a plaque undergoing acute fissuring. The basis of the crescendo form of unstable angina is the unstable plaque (33,34).

Pathogenesis of symptoms in 'thrombotic' unstable angina
There are several putative mechanisms of intermittent ischaemia in patients with an active plaque fissure and associated mural thrombus.

Figure 2.13
Type I stenosis seen on (left) angiography (*post mortem*). The narrowed segment has a smooth outline and there is no intraluminal filling defect. The histology of the plaque (right) shows an eccentric lesion with no evidence of thrombosis.

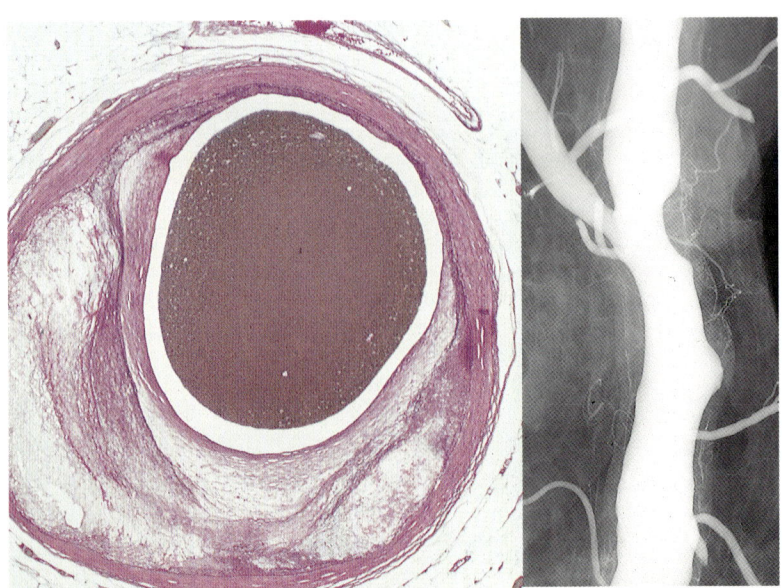

Figure 2.14
Angiogram of Type II stenosis *post mortem*. The stenotic segment has an irregular outline and there are filling defects due to thrombosis within the lumen.

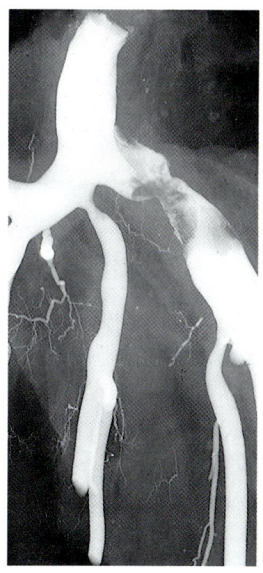

Figure 2.15
Histology (transverse section) of a plaque which has undergone fissuring. There is a defect in the plaque cap which has been torn at its lateral insertion into the more normal intima. The mass of thrombus has one lobe inside the plaque and another within the lumen, and the two are joined through the fissure.

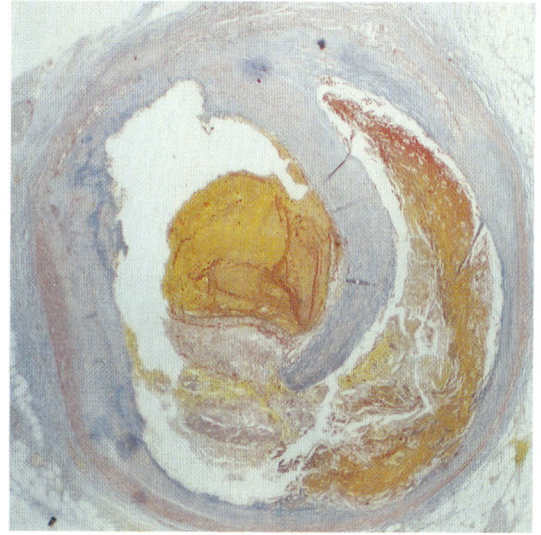

Intermittent complete occlusion by thrombus within the lumen. This mechanism has been demonstrated by angiography in patients who ultimately progress to persistent occlusion with infarction. There is no doubt that the thrombus within the lumen is labile, waxing and waning in size over short periods of time (35).

Intermittent distal embolization. The thrombus which forms within the fissure site has a superficial coating of platelets on the luminal surface; from this layer, clumps of platelets embolize into the myocardium. Post-mortem studies show these microemboli to be associated with microscopic foci of myocardial necrosis and occur in up to 50% of patients with unstable angina (32,36). A number of clinical studies in unstable angina have shown that episodes of pain are associated with evidence of enhanced platelet activation (37,38).

Intermittent arterial spasm at the site of fissuring and/or intermittent increase of resistance in the distal myocardial microvascular bed. The evidence for alterations in vascular tone being responsible for the intermittent ischaemia in unstable angina with plaque rupture is mostly theoretical. Many unstable plaques are eccentric with a potential for local spasm. Thrombus within the plaque releases a plethora of potent vasoconstrictors which may act either locally or on the distal vascular bed. Vasodilatory drugs are clinically effective, which supports the view that spasm has a role in the production of symptoms.

Progression of Type II lesions
The clinical history and angiograms of patients with unstable angina show that active fissuring and mural thrombus occur for periods of up to three weeks (39) but, ultimately, the lesion either progresses to form a persistent occlusion, explaining the risk of acute myocardial infarction, or the fissure resolves and restabilizes, leaving a patent vessel. The mechanism of resolution to vessel patency is by smooth muscle proliferation which seals the fissure, and the irregular outline of the stenosis becomes smooth due to an overlay of new collagen. A small proportion of lesions develops a small cratered ulcer with overhanging edges, indicating that the whole of the plaque contents has been evacuated (40) and the cap totally destroyed. Persistent ulcerated plaques in which exposed thrombus remains in the base, however, do not appear to be common findings in the coronary arteries, unlike in the carotid arteries where they are a source of microemboli and cerebral transient ischaemic attacks.

Vasospasm and unstable angina
In normal coronary arteries, the cross-sectional area of the lumen is controlled by the tone of the circumferential medial smooth muscle cells. Intimal smooth muscle cells are arranged haphazardly and are involved in the synthesis of connective tissue matrix rather than in contraction. The media is avascular in normal arteries and does not contain nerve fibres; these are, however, present in abundance in the adjacent adventitia.

Smooth muscle tone is influenced by endothelium-derived relaxing factor (EDRF) (41) as well as by a variety of neuropeptides released from nerve endings in the adventitia. These mediators diffuse into the media to act directly on smooth muscle cells. There is experimental evidence that EDRF is continually produced and acts upon the epicardial arteries probably by adjusting the vascular tone and luminal size to accommodate flow increase and reduce shear stress. Normal human coronary arteries dilate on exercise and after infusion of acetylcholine (42). The increase in flow itself is mediated by a fall in resistance within the distal vascular bed. Many vasodilatory substances act indirectly by initiating EDRF production; acetyl-choline, for example, is a vasodilator in the presence of an intact endothelial surface but, if the endothelium is absent, a direct vasoconstrictor effect on medial smooth muscle cells is unmasked. EDRF appears to be nitric oxide produced by catabolism of arginine and released from the abluminal side of the endothelial cell (43). Adventitial nerves release a number of vasoconstrictors including noradrenaline and neuropeptide Y as well as vasodilators, such as substance P and calcitonin gene-related peptide (CGRP). The precise balance between these factors and which are predominant in determining normal coronary vessel tone is uncertain. Normal tonal variations occur within a range of up to a 20% reduction in the length of a smooth muscle cell, but hypercontraction may occlude even a morphologically normal artery. The term 'spasm' is often applied to this extreme degree of medial contraction (44).

Prinzmetal's variant angina is the result of coronary artery spasm (45). In some patients, the coronary artery tree is angiographically normal between episodes of spasm; in others, however, although the relaxed vessel shows no stenosis, spasm occurs at specific sites and the outline of the vessel is slightly irregular. Necropsy studies are infrequent, but suggest that at least some patients with Prinzmetal's angina have diffuse non-stenosing coronary atheroma (45). In some patients, however, there is no angiographic evidence of atherosclerosis, yet spasm occurs at the same parts over many years. This form of angina, therefore, is also seen as part of a general abnormality of smooth muscle tone linked with evidence of abnormal tone in other sites, for example, migraine.

There is a growing body of evidence of abnormal vasomotor responses in atherosclerotic coronary arteries. In patients with ischaemic heart disease, the response of angiographically normal segments of artery to an infusion of acetylcholine is to constrict rather than dilate (42). This paradoxical response suggests that the direct action of acetylcholine on smooth muscle is overriding the indirect effects of EDRF. In patients with ischaemic heart disease, the normal increase in the diameter of epicardial coronary arteries on exercise or with a cold pressor test is lost (46). In animals in which atheroma has been induced, the vasodilator response to acetylcholine is lost as in in-vitro responses seen in man of coronary arteries from transplanted hearts (47). The hypothesis has therefore evolved that there is widespread endothelial dysfunction in atheromatous vessels, particularly with regard to EDRF production, which accords with the morphological evidence that ultrastructural endothelial damage is common over apparently intact plaques. Regenerated endothelium does not regain its potential for EDRF production for a long period of time (48), and it must be borne in mind that, in atherosclerotic arteries, there may be continuous endothelial regeneration.

Normal variations in medial tone may significantly influence blood flow at points where there is concomitant high-grade fixed stenosis wherein the eccentric plaque allows retention of an arc of normal vessel wall in relation to the residual lumen. It has been calculated (15) that in order for tone variation to influence flow, there must be a fixed stenosis of a greater than 50% diameter reduction with a 60°arc of normal media. Spasm, however, may alter flow at lesions with a less severe degree of fixed stenosis.

Cases of sudden onset unstable angina have been clearly described in which an abnormal vasomotor response at the site of an eccentric stenosis was responsible for symptoms. In the best documented case (45), symptoms were clearly related to an eccentric stenosis in the right coronary artery where the luminal area was reduced from 1.5 sq mm to 0.16 sq mm by an infusion of adrenaline with a marked increase in resistance to flow across the lesion. The lesion was excised at the time of cardiac surgery to insert a saphenous vein graft and was confirmed as an eccentric plaque with a lipid pool, but no evidence of plaque rupture. Major intraluminal thrombosis was absent, but microthrombus formation on the endothelial surface was clearly seen. In experimental arterial injury, vasospasm and platelet deposition are closely linked (49).

Other cases of unstable angina have been reported in which eccentric stenosis was associated with an adventitial inflammatory cell infiltrate, including basophilic mast cells and eosinophils. The hypothesis put forward is that adventitial nerves are influenced or damaged by this inflammatory cell infiltrate, leading to an imbalance of nerve-mediated constriction and dilatation (50).

There are several possible causes of altered vasomotor responses at sites of eccentric stenosis (see Box opposite).

Although firm evidence for any of these mechanisms is not yet available, the concept of altered tonal responses in atheromatous vessels is well established.

An overview of angina

It is currently accepted that a patient with angina may have any possible permutation of fixed stenosis, dynamic stenosis (varying with medial tone) and intraluminal thrombosis. Stable exertional angina and ischaemia related only to a demonstrable increase in myocardial oxygen demand is due to a fixed stenosis. Patients in whom there is additional evidence of transient ischaemia disproportionate to oxygen demand are considered to have an element of variable or dynamic stenosis superimposing a fixed stenosis. Unstable angina is due to major thrombosis or spasm, or both. The wide spectrum of clinical severity of unstable angina is partly responsible for the uncertainty over the dominant mechanism. Patients at the severe end of

A functional abnormality of EDRF production;

A functional endothelial abnormality plus minor structural damage and microthrombosis affecting release of platelet-derived constrictors;

A reduced response to EDRF because of intimal thickening passively blocking access to the medial smooth muscle cell;

Increased neutralization of EDRF within the intima by plasma constituents, such as haemoglobin;

Adventitial inflammation;

Increased medial smooth muscle sensitivity to vasoconstrictors.

the spectrum, seen in specialized units, are those who have angiography, have a risk of dying and eventually are submitted to post-mortem examination. The preponderance of thrombosis and the importance of plaque fissuring reported in these cases may not apply to patients with milder symptoms, who are neither investigated nor die, although thrombosis or spasm may be present. More information may be derived from knowing which therapy is effective in relieving symptoms but, in practice, many patients receive a cocktail of drugs to cover a broad spectrum of eventualities.

A further grey area surrounds the mechanism of short episodic periods of transient ischaemia, which may occur over many months in patients with a stable exertional angina or after a healed myocardial infarct. These episodes may, in part, be related to an increase in heart rate and myocardial oxygen demand, but there is compelling evidence that the degree of ischaemia is out of proportion to these increases, and a decrease in coronary blood flow must be present. The mechanism for this reduction or failure to increase flow in response to demand is not known. A rational hypothesis is that there is either vasoconstriction in the epicardial arteries or a redistribution of blood by selective constriction of intramyocardial vessels. That endothelial dysfunction is responsible for these tonal abnormalities and for transient ischaemia in coronary atherosclerosis is very appealing and, if proven to be true, would indicate that transient ischaemia, often short-lived and silent as regards pain, identifies those patients with progressive atherosclerosis.

Acute myocardial infarction

Arterial lesions

Clinically, the term 'acute myocardial infarction' usually refers to regional myocardial necrosis, either transmural or non-transmural (confined to the subendocardium). The regional distribution of necrosis mirrors the territory supplied by the various coronary arteries or their major branches, and suggests that an arterial lesion is responsible for the infarction. In the past, there has been controversy over the exact nature of this lesion, in particular the role of thrombosis in the subtending artery. Sequential angiography has resolved the argument in living patients as it allows flow in the artery to be assessed over short intervals of time.

Many studies have now been published, following the seminal work of Marcus DeWood (51), Stadius and colleagues (52) and Bertrand and co-workers (53). In addition, further studies are reporting on the influence of thrombolytic therapy on the occluded artery (54,55).

In the early phase (one to six hours), there is a high (over 80%) incidence of total occlusion of the artery supplying the region of infarction.

A proportion of these arteries subsequently spontaneously reopen. By the tenth day, as many as 50% of the vessels have antegrade flow re-established.

The use of fibrinolytic drugs increases the proportion in and speed with which antegrade flow is re-established in occluded arteries. In some series, over 80% of occluded arteries were reopened, although others reported less striking success.

As antegrade flow is restored, intraluminal filling defects are revealed which slowly diminish in size.

As antegrade flow is restored, in many cases a Type II stenosis is revealed.

Retrospective analysis of previous angiograms shows that occlusion does not inevitably develop at sites of previous high-grade stenosis (56,57). It is, therefore, impossible to predict the site of a future infarct from earlier angiograms.

The conclusions derived from these data are that thrombosis is a major element in occlusion and is a very dynamic process. This does not exclude the possibility that spasm at the site of obstruction or impedance to flow in the distal vascular bed within the myocardium may reduce flow and, thus, favour thrombus formation. The thrombotic process in the artery has been shown in radiolabelling studies of both platelets and fibrinogen to continue after the inception of infarction (58,59). Similar studies, however, have also demonstrated that there is a more proximal nidus of thrombus which is not labelled and, therefore, predates the onset of myocardial infarction (60).

Plaque events precipitating thrombosis
Pathology plays a valuable role in describing the structure of the intima underlying major coronary thrombi and, in particular, the events in atheromatous plaques which initiate thrombosis. Reconstruction of plaques underlying thrombi related to acute regional infarction shows that the majority (75%) have undergone deep intimal injury with fissuring (rupture) while 25% are not related to fissuring, but are due to more superficial injury with diffuse endothelial loss.

Types of myocardial infarction in man
Animal models of infarction in which a coronary artery is ligated, causing virtually instantaneous occlusion, are widely used as analogues of the situation in man. These simple models, predominantly undertaken in the dog, have established that necrosis begins in the subendocardial zone and spreads outward as a wave front to the epicardial surface over a period of six hours. The removal of the ligature to allow reperfusion after periods of up to six hours of total occlusion prevents extension of the infarction to become transmural, but the lateral border of the necrosis is determined at the time of occlusion and is not altered by reperfusion. Six hours is a short period of time in terms of tissue reaction, and the histological appearances of the myocardium is uniform throughout the area of necrosis in these experimental infarcts.

Although the disease in man is more complex than in this simple animal model, there is no reason to suppose that the basic principles established in the ligation models are not the same. In man, there is a spectrum in the structure of regional infarcts which ranges from lesions in which the necrosis is of uniform age (Figures 2.16 & 2.17) to those which appear to have been built up by the coalescence of smaller areas of necrosis of widely differing ages (Figure 2.18). It is reasonable to suppose that the latter are the result of episodes of intermittent occlusion occurring over a period of days. This stuttering onset in some infarcts in man is supported by the prodromal symptoms experienced by many patients prior to a fully developed infarction and by angiographic studies in patients undergoing infarction (61). The practical difficulty thus created for clinicians is to define precisely when infarction can be said to begin in man and will, at best, be inexact.

Figure 2.16
Regional transmural infarction is best demonstrated at necropsy by the loss of dehydrogenase activity in the necrotic muscle. Normal myocardium stains purple when treated with succinate and nitro blue tetrazolium due to its enzyme activity. In the short-axis transection of the left ventricle, there is a transmural area of pale infarcted myocardium on the posterior wall of the left ventricle, involving the posteromedial papillary muscle and posterior third of the interventricular septum, corresponding exactly to the region of myocardium supplied by the right coronary artery. On the lateral wall of the left ventricle lies the dense white fibrous tissue of an old scar.

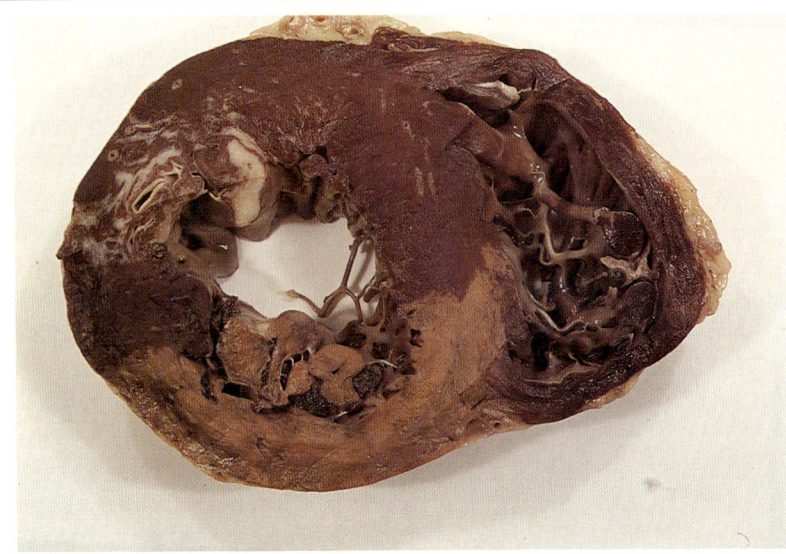

Figure 2.17
A regional non-transmural infarction is present in an identical distribution to that in Figure 2.16. There is a zone of subpericardial normal muscle in which enzyme activity was retained.

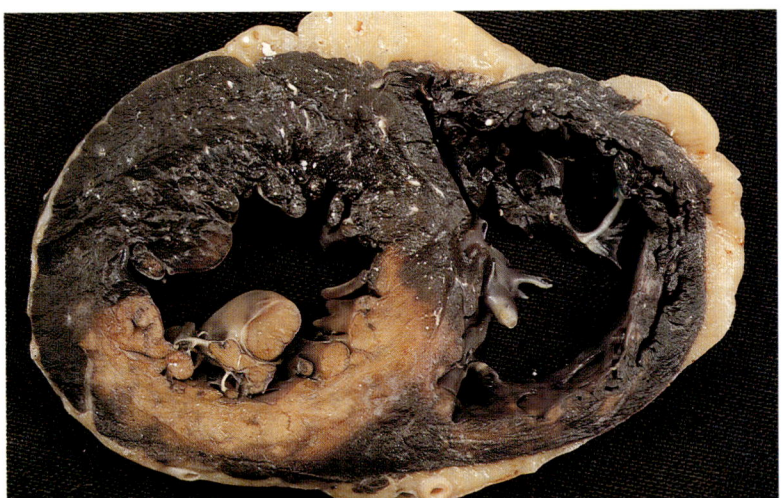

Figure 2.18
Detail of a non-transmural infarction which is made up of smaller focal areas of different age and, thus, shows considerable variation in colour. There are areas of no enzyme activity while other areas show reduced colour intensity.

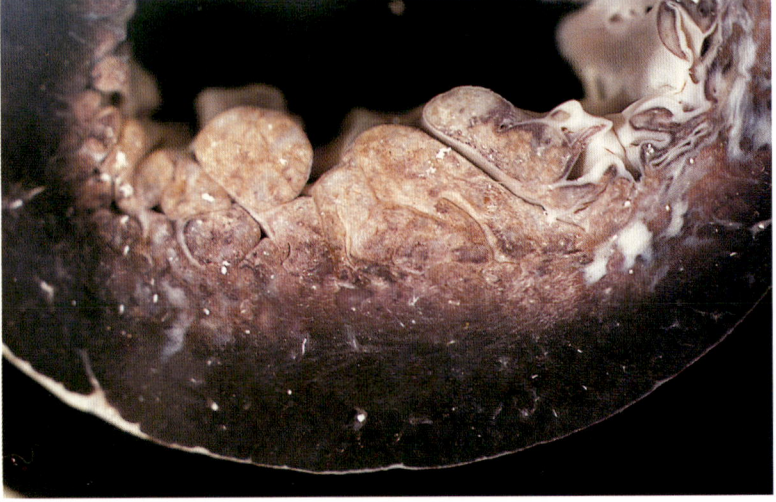

Transmural versus non-transmural regional infarction in man
The concordance between Q *versus* non-Q wave infarction on electrocardiography, and transmural *versus* non-transmural infarction at subsequent post-mortem examination, has been shown to be far from perfect (62). In spite of this, the angiographic factors associated with non-Q wave infarction in living subjects (63) are very similar to those found in post-mortem angiographic studies of non-transmural regional infarction (Table 2.1). This lends support to the concept that a non-Q wave infarct is not transmural. Transmural and non-transmural infarctions are not in reality clearly distinguishable. At one extreme, there are infarcts in which the endocardial and epicardial extent of necrosis is identical and the infarct is transmural throughout. At the other extreme, there are infarcts which are wholly non-transmural and the pericardial surface is not involved at any point. Between these extremes, however, are infarcts of any possible ratio between endocardial and epicardial extent, with the former always being larger. In an infarct with an epicardial area of only 10% of the endocardial area, the transmural component is small and may not be appreciated unless multiple ECG leads are used or multiple planes examined at autopsy.

Angiographic studies in life (63) show that, in non-Q wave infarction at any particular time interval after the onset of pain, there is a far higher frequency of arterial patency than with Q-wave infarction (64). Collateral development is better in patients with non-Q rather than Q wave infarction, as confirmed in necropsy studies comparing non-transmural with transmural infarction (65). Pathological studies show that the proportion of patients with non-transmural infarction who have filling of the artery distal to the site of thrombosis is far higher than in transmural infarction (Table 2.1). Filling of the distal vessel may occur either *via* antegrade flow over the thrombus or *via* collaterals.

Table 2.1 Coronary artery status in regional infarction: Mural versus non-transmural

	Transmural	Non-transmural
Antegrade flow (mural thrombus) Distal vessel filled	8 (29%)	13 (65%)
No antegrade flow (occlusive thrombus) Distal filling via collaterals	7 (25%)	7 (35%)
No antegrade flow (occlusive thrombus) No distal filling	13 (46%)	0
Total numbers (%)	28 (100%)	20 (100%)

> Regional non-transmural infarction indicates that flow to the subepicardial zone has been maintained either by restoration of antegrade flow or by previously established collateral flow.

In man, the stimulus for the development of collaterals is high-grade stenosis leading to a difference in perfusion pressure between two adjacent myocardial segments. An ideal situation is where previous high-grade stenosis has invoked such florid collateral flow that no infarction develops following thrombosis of the artery supplying the area. Pathological studies (19) suggest that up to 23% of total occlusions do not cause infarction because of extensive previously established collateral flow.

The structure of infarcts in man is therefore very much more complex than the simple experimental models in current use (see Box).

> Many arterial occlusions in man are not instantaneous, but are initially intermittent over several hours or days.
>
> Collateral flow between adjacent perfusion beds may have been previously established.

Infarct size in man depends on many variables acting on the basic anatomical arrangement which determines the area of myocardium at risk. The largest transmural infarcts result from instantaneous occlusion of arteries supplying large territories in which there has been no previous high-grade stenosis, no history of angina and no collateral flow. Occlusion of, for example, the left anterior descending artery above the first septal branch in the absence of established collaterals, leads to loss of 40% of the left ventricular muscle mass, a transmural anteroseptal infarct, and a very high incidence of cardiogenic shock and septal rupture. The absence of collateral flow is a major factor in determining whether the infarct will be transmural and, thus, indirectly determines whether infarct expansion, rupture or aneurysm formation will occur (66,67).

Non-regional forms of myocardial necrosis
Myocardial necrosis not spatially related to a specific coronary artery or branch is the result of a failure of overall myocardial perfusion and has no relationship to coronary thrombosis other than indirectly in some instances. Prolonged hypotension from any cause leads to underperfusion of the entire subendocardial zone of the left ventricle, including the papillary muscles, resulting in circumferential subendocardial necrosis, which is

sometimes referred to as laminar infarction. Ventricular hypertrophy enhances susceptibility to this form of necrosis. Cardiogenic shock is often complicated by diffuse subendocardial necrosis superimposed on an initial regional transmural infarct.

Infarct extension, expansion and ventricular remodelling
The terms 'extension' and 'expansion' have very precise and different meanings (Figure 2.19), but are often used interchangeably. Infarct extension refers to additional myocardial necrosis superimposing at a later date on the original area of infarction. The term is used in clinical practise to explain the development of more widespread electrocardiographic changes or a diminishing left ventricular function in a patient with an acute infarct; in this case, the term encompasses two very different processes: In one, a non-transmural infarct extends to become a full-thickness infarct, but the lateral border does not change. This is due to reocclusion of the subtending artery before the development of collateral flow into the epicardial zone. In the other form of extension, the new necrosis is not regional, but develops as a circumferential subendocardial layer throughout the left ventricle; this is due to a decline in overall myocardial perfusion. The majority of patients with cardiogenic shock who are examined *post mortem* have this form of infarct extension and it is likely that there is a relentless downward spiral of falling myocardial per-

Figure 2.19
Comparison of the different processes of infarct extension and infarct expansion.

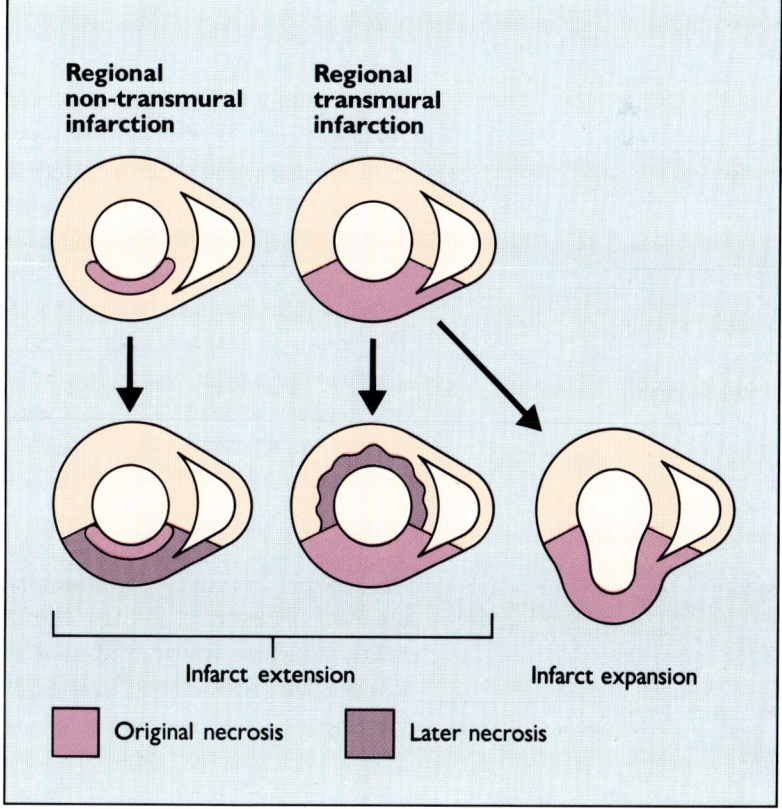

fusion causing subendocardial necrosis which, in turn, results in a further decline in ventricular function and myocardial perfusion.

Infarct expansion (68) refers to 'stretching' of the area of necrosis so that its external dimensions increase; this is usually associated with wall-thinning, but without the development of new necrosis. Expansion occurs either by the sliding and slippage of adjacent dead myocytes in relation to each other or by the muscle bundles tearing apart within the infarct. The latter may be associated with a ragged tear of a centimetre or more in the endocardium. Replacement of such an expanded infarct by fibrosis consolidates the new shape and prevents the return to more normal ventricular dimensions. Non-transmural infarcts do not, with rare exceptions, expand. Apart from the area of infarction itself, expanding dilatation of the left ventricle as a whole may become fixed after a relatively short time. It is uncertain whether this is due to an increase in connective tissue matrix or a change in myocyte configuration.

Reparative processes in myocardial infarction
The ultimate fate of necrotic myocytes is removal by macrophages, with the ingress of new capillaries and fibroblasts ('organization') leading to the deposition of collagen and the formation of a myocardial scar. An acute polymorphonuclear response is present in the blood vessels and interstitial spaces in the first 12 hours, but is rapidly replaced by macrophage activity.

The sequential timing of this process has been established in animal models of infarction, but the more complex process of infarction in man prohibits a precise determination of the onset of infarction using the histology.

In large regional transmural infarcts, the centre of the lesion is completely avascular due to blockage of small vessels by polymorphs and/or hypoxic endothelial swelling, resulting in necrosis of both myocytes and the stroma, including blood vessels. These changes are a factor in preventing reperfusion of areas of established infarction.

Organization of the infarct, that is, replacement by fibrosis, only arises when the necrotic area is invaded by capillaries and fibroblasts from the viable tissues at the margin of the infarct; often, several weeks may pass before the centre is reached. Incarcerated dead myocytes with a recognizable structure may be present for up to several months in the infarct centre. In contrast, if an infarct is the result of coalescence of necrotic areas of different ages, the stroma often survives. Internal organization and replacement by fibrosis may be very rapid and is typical of non-transmural infarction.

Complications of myocardial infarction

Cardiac arrest due to ventricular fibrillation induced by acute ischaemia is discussed in detail in Chapter 3. From the pathologists' viewpoint, there has been a significant change in hospital findings at necropsy of acute infarction. Up to 1970, arrhythmic deaths in hospital were commonplace, and bore no clear relationship to infarct size; pathologists often saw patients who should have survived an infarct as no more than 10% of the left ventricular mass was involved. Today, such cases are virtually confined to patients who were not admitted to hospital because of their stoical acceptance of pain, a failure to realize its significance or silent infarction. Cardiogenic shock has become the major cause of in-hospital mortality from acute infarction.

Cardiogenic shock

Cardiogenic shock is due to loss of a major proportion (more than 30%) of the left ventricular mass, and is associated with sudden occlusion of large coronary arteries, such as the proximal left anterior descending branch, in cases where there has been no previous angina nor stenosis nor collateral development in the region. Often superimposing on the regional component of infarction is a diffuse circumferential subendocardial necrosis as myocardial perfusion diminishes. A small subgroup of patients with cardiogenic shock do not have regional acute necrosis, but appear to develop diffuse subendocardial necrosis in a ventricle which has had extensive previous infarction as small focal areas of scarring throughout the myocardium, rather than large discrete regional infarcts.

Left ventricular mural thrombi in acute infarction

The majority of mural thrombi related to acute infarction are due to akinetic segments of myocardium enlarging the apical area of stasis normally present in the left ventricle (Figure 2.20). Stasis is regarded as the dominant pathogenetic feature, although inflammatory mediators released from the infarct zone may have a subsidiary role (69). The risk of thrombosis is directly related to infarct size and confined to transmural infarction. Large anteroapical infarcts (peak creatine phosphokinase concentration greater than 2000 units) have a 50% incidence of mural thrombi and, in 10%, systemic emboli occur (70).

Myocardial rupture

Most pathological series (71) report that up to 10% of in-hospital mortality of acute infarction is due to rupture of the ventricular myocardium into the pericardial sac, resulting in death from tamponade. There are several forms of rupture with different pathophysiological mechanisms and time schedules before the onset of pain. A consistent finding is that external cardiac rupture is more common, in relation to the number of

Figure 2.20
An acute anteroapical infarct which has expanded. The resulting acute aneurysm has filled with ante-mortem thrombus.

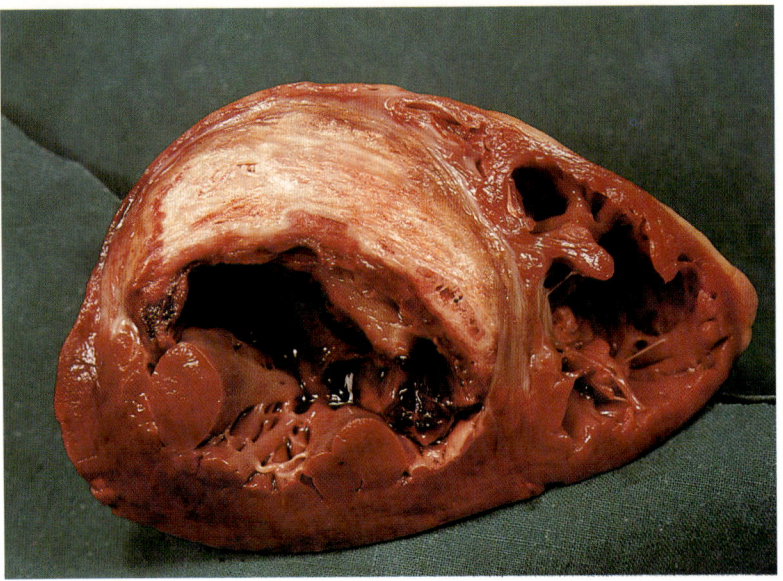

infarcts overall, in older women than in men (72). A putative factor is infiltration of the myocardium by adipose tissue which occurs in older women. External rupture always indicates a transmural infarct, and a clinical advantage of non-transmural, rather than transmural, infarction is the absence of risk of either external or internal rupture and aneurysm formation.

There is a form of external rupture (73) which occurs within 24 hours of the onset of pain, often before it is possible to identify easily the infarct by naked-eye examination at necropsy. The rupture occurs as a slit at the margin of viable and non-viable tissue (Figures 2.21 & 2.22) in an infarct in which there has been no change in configuration of the left ventricle. Inflammation in the pericardium adjacent to the external aperture is absent, and the appearances suggest a sudden catastrophic event.

Another form of rupture occurs much later after the onset of pain (four to seven days). The infarct is expanded (74) and bulges outward as an aneurysm with a thinned wall. Infarction is at the stage where soft, yellow, necrotic material is contained in the centre of the infarct. Rupture may occur at the apex of the ventricular bulge or there may be an endocardial tear through which the soft centre of the infarct is evacuated by a haematoma rupturing outward at another site. Acute pericarditis over the external surface near the point of rupture is common, suggesting that long-term slow leakage of blood precedes the final rupture.

Ventricular septal rupture
The mechanism of septal rupture is identical to that which occurs in external rupture. Both anteroseptal and posteroseptal infarcts may be complicated by rupture (75); the former leads to a defect which may enter the right ventricle anteriorly at

Figure 2.21
Point of ventricular rupture into the pericardial sac at 24 hours post-onset of pain. The infarcted area is not expanded and there is no pericarditis.

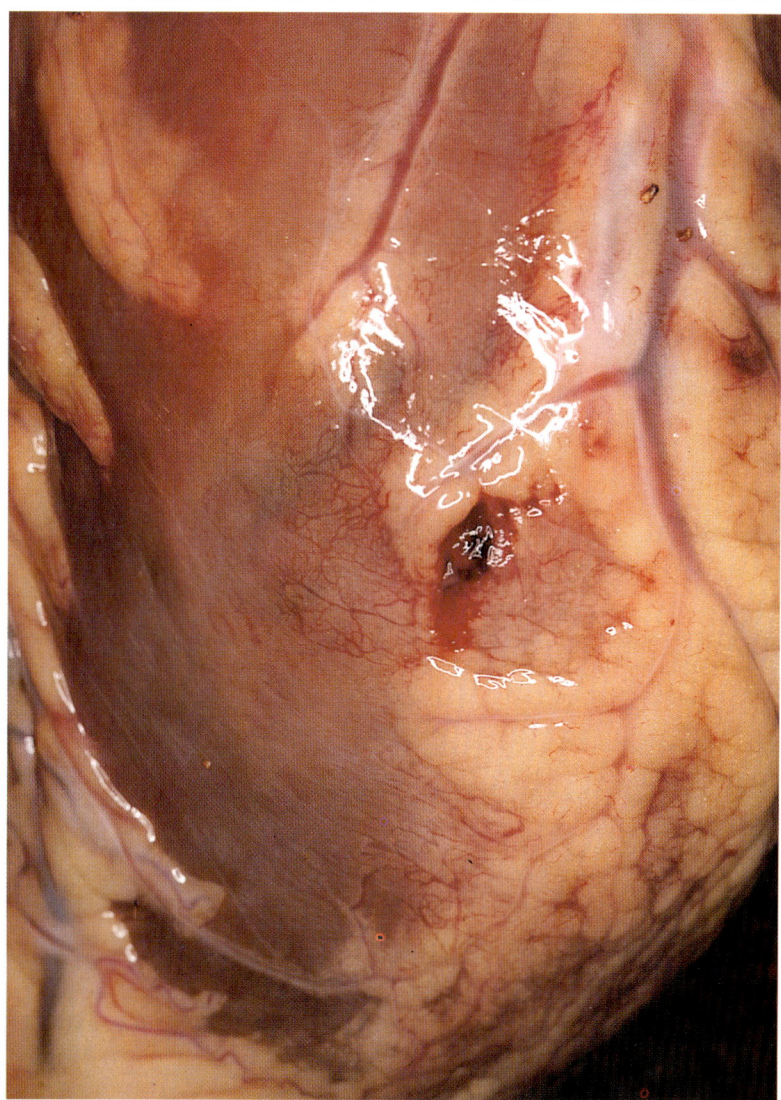

Figure 2.22
Short-axis transection of early rupture of a lateral infarct which, at this stage, is not easily distinguished by naked-eye examination. A track joins the endocardium to the epicardium at the margin of infarct. Expansion is absent.

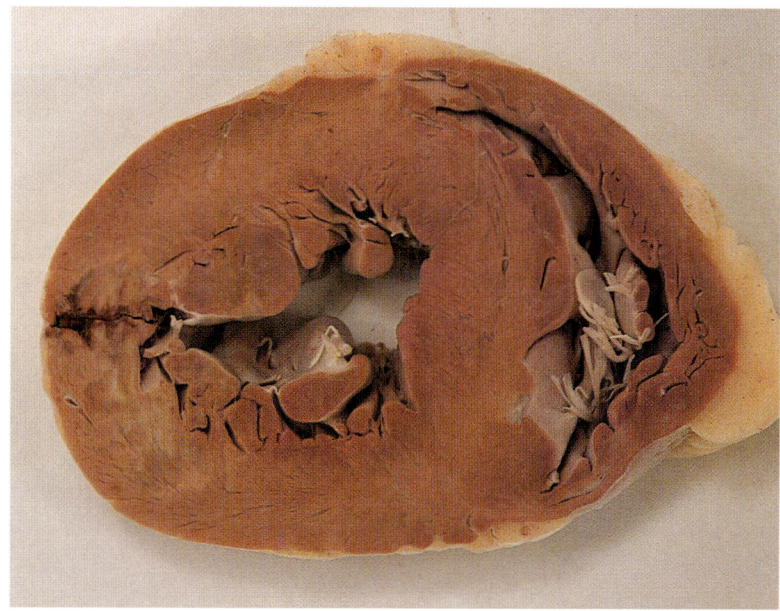

any point from the apex to the outflow tract, and is almost always associated with a very proximal left anterior descending branch occlusion in the absence of previously established collateral flow (Figure 2.23). Posteroinferior septal infarcts enter the right ventricle high on the posterior aspect of the septum, close to the tricuspid valve, and have a strong association with aneurysm formation on the posterior left ventricular wall. The septal tears range from slits to ragged tears of several square centimeters surrounded by necrotic myocardium. In patients who survive without surgical closure, the defect ultimately becomes a smooth rounded hole surrounded by fibrous tissue. A study of 500 consecutive in-hospital acute infarct deaths (71) showed 11 examples (2.2%) of such ventricular septal defects.

Figure 2.23
Long-axis view of an anteroseptal acute infarct which has expanded and thinned. It had also contained a mural thrombus within the apical portion of the left ventricle. The septum has ruptured into the right ventricle at the apex of the bulging infarct.

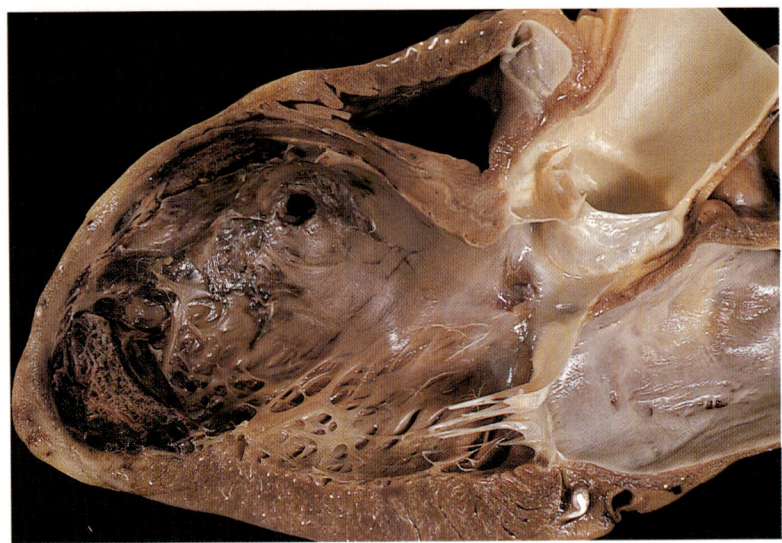

Ischaemic ventricular aneurysms
The pathological definition of a ventricular aneurysm is a local external bulge protruding from the external surface of the ventricle, but there is no generally accepted definition of the size of the bulge. There is even more variation in the clinical use of the term, particularly in the setting of acute infarction where localized akinesia in the systolic phase may be termed an aneurysm with a minimal degree of external bulging. For these reasons, the reported incidence of ischaemic aneurysms ranges from 4 to 40% after an acute infarct (76).

Pathological examination of chronic aneurysms resulting from ischaemic heart disease show a range of morphology from those with a wide neck to those with a very narrow neck leading to a large external space, and including all gradations in between (Figures 2.24-2.26).

Three mechanisms lead to the formation of aneurysms subsequent to an acute transmural inarction (see Box).

Figure 2.24
An apical left ventricular aneurysm with a wide neck which does not contain thrombus.

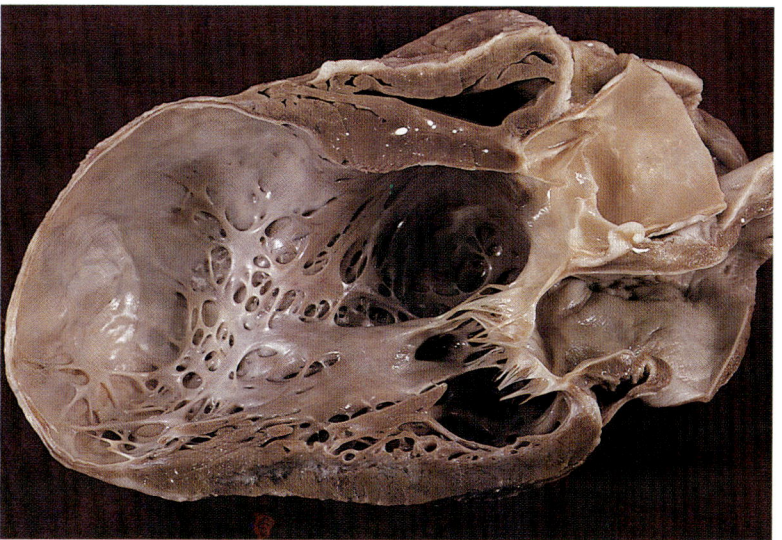

Expansion of the acute infarct may form an aneurysmal bulge within two to four days. Subsequent fibrosis makes the aneurysm permanent.

A large infarct becomes organized and replaced by fibrosis, but later aneurysm formation occurs within seven days and before there is sufficient tensile strength in the scar to resist systolic pressure in the ventricular cavity.

There is a 'near-miss' external rupture in which a haematoma forms beneath the pericardium. Fibrosis of the pericardium over the haematoma leads ultimately to a large sac external to the ventricle, but connected to the ventricular cavity by a very small neck at the site of the original myocardial rupture.

Aneurysms thought to arise from 'near-miss' external rupture are often termed 'pseudoaneurysms' because the wall of the sac is not myocardial tissue, but pericardial. In reality, however, determination of the exact mechanism leading to the formation of a given aneurysm is difficult without necropsy and histological examination of the sac wall (77). Studies in which this has been done show that some aneurysms with narrow necks do comprise a wall derived from myocardium and not pericardium and, thus, are true aneurysms (78).

Clinical evidence suggests that many aneurysms develop very early after the onset of acute infarction, and the role of infarct expansion is currently regarded as the most important factor involved; no new aneurysms arise after three months (79). It is thought that aneurysms with narrow necks and large external sacs, by implication 'false', have a greater propensity to late rupture than diffuse aneurysms (80). This may be true, but the evidence so far is anecdotal and based on case reports. Diffuse aneurysms with wide necks, however, have a thicker external wall, so the risk of late rupture would appear to be minimal.

Mural thrombus (Figures 2.25 & 2.26) is present in approximately 50% of chronic ischaemic aneurysms, but no particular factor of shape or age has been identified to be predictive of its presence or absence. Thromboembolic phenomenon are found *post mortem* in approximately 30% of ischaemic aneurysms; although recognized as a major clinical risk, studies in living patients record an incidence of only 5% (81). Calcification in the aneurysm wall is common and can often be seen on radiography outlining the sac. The degree of fibroelastic endocardial thickening varies widely within and at the margins of the aneurysmal sac. A very thick endocardial lining (Type I) is associated with a low incidence of thrombus formation, but with a high frequency of recurrent ventricular tachycardia while, conversely, a thin lining (Type II) is associated with a higher incidence of mural thrombus and a lower frequency of ventricular tachycardia (82).

Figure 2.25
Posterior ischaemic aneurysm with a thin fibrous wall. The diameter of the external sac is larger than that of the neck by a ratio of 1.4:1. The sac contains thrombus.

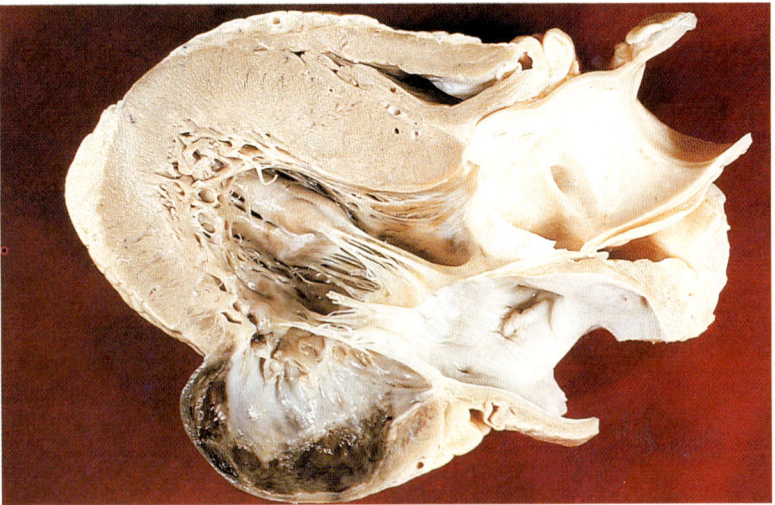

Papillary muscle infarction

Acute infarction of the posteromedial papillary muscle group occurs in up to 40% of posteroinferior infarcts and is less common (approximately 15%) in the anterolateral papillary muscle group in association with anterior infarction. The lower frequency in the anterolateral group reflects the origin of the blood supply from the left circumflex artery *via* the left marginal branch, which is not a common site of thrombosis. The sequelae of acute papillary muscle infarction range from catastrophic sudden mitral regurgitation through chronic mild mitral regurgitation to no haemodynamic effect.

Figure 2.26
Ischaemic 'pseudoaneurysm' in which the external sac is very large (22 cm) and opens into the cavity of the left ventricle by an aperture which is less than a centimetre across. The sac contains a large quantity of laminated thrombus.

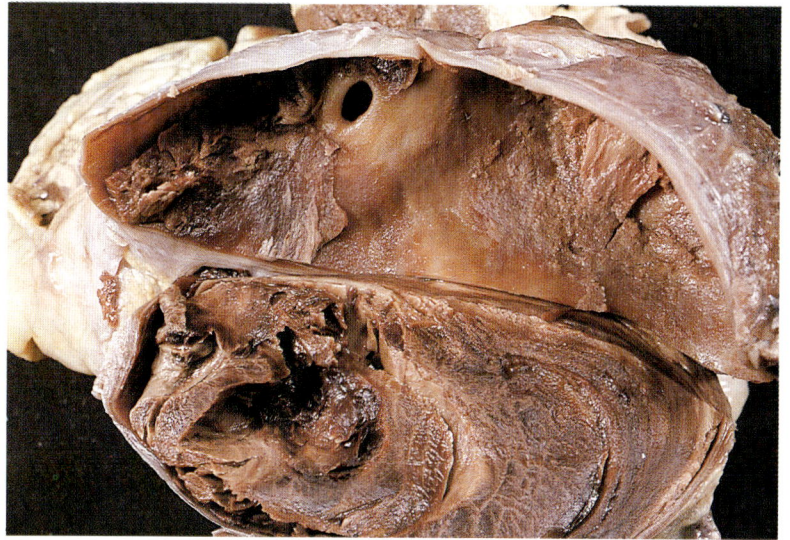

Papillary muscle rupture (83,84) is the result of tearing of the soft infarcted papillary muscle. This may be complete avulsion of the whole of a papillary muscle at the base, close to its insertion into the ventricular wall, to avulsion of only the tip of a papillary muscle with a small number of its attached chordae. The chordae are avascular and not involved and, thus, do not primarily rupture in ischaemia. Acute regurgitation ranges in degree from catastrophic, when the whole of a papillary muscle stump crosses and recrosses the mitral orifice (Figure 2.27), to relatively minor. Papillary muscle rupture is rare. A detailed in-hospital autopsy study of 500 consecutive fatal acute infarcts (71) revealed only six cases (1.2%).

Figure 2.27
Complete avulsion of a papillary muscle due to infarction. The valve is viewed from the left atrium which, after prolapse across the mitral orifice, now contains the papillary muscle.

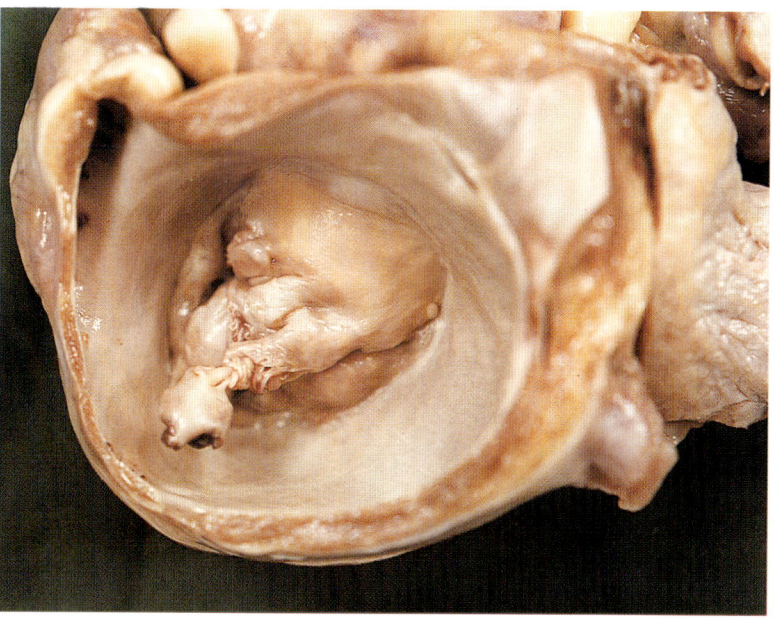

Chronic mitral regurgitation following acute infarction is due to fixed elongation of an intact papillary muscle. As with aneurysm formation, it may be that elongation of the papillary muscle occurs very early and, subsequently, becomes permanent after fibrosis.

Sudden ischaemic death

Seventy percent of all sudden natural deaths (less than or equal to six hours after onset of symptoms in the last episode) is due to ischaemic heart disease (85). If sudden is defined as less than one hour from onset of symptoms, there is no alteration to this percentage rate but, if the temporal definition is extended to 24 hours, the figure decreases. Four times more men than women die suddenly from ischaemic heart disease and, in women, ischaemic heart disease is not the most common cause of sudden natural death. Many studies of sudden ischaemic death show that, in approximately 50% of cases, death is the presenting feature and the patient was unaware of having coronary atheroma.

The pathological basis of the sudden occurrence of death in patients with longstanding coronary atheroma was once controversial; today, both pathological and clinical data of resuscitated cases of out-of-hospital cardiac arrest indicate a failure to appreciate the existence of two separate mechanisms. In both, however, the final common pathway is ventricular fibrillation.

One of the mechanisms involves a new acute vascular event with thrombosis, and the arterial pathology is identical to that of abrupt-onset unstable angina. Arteriography at necropsy shows either Type II stenosis with intraluminal thrombus or a complete thrombotic occlusion based on plaque fissuring (12). There is a high incidence of acute ischaemic damage in the myocardium distal to the acute vascular lesion ranging from microscopic focal necrosis to transmural infarction. The predicted outcome, had these patients survived, would be that some would develop ECG or enzymatic changes of acute infarction while, in others, the plaque fissure would resolve with minimal myocardial damage. Clinical study of resuscitated cases only detects those with more major myocardial damage.

With the other mechanism leading to sudden ischaemic death, necropsy does not reveal a new acute vascular lesion, but there is healed myocardial infarction, often in association with left ventricular hypertrophy. These patients have advanced stenosis in two or three major coronary vessels.

In the first group of sudden ischaemic deaths, arrhythmias arise because of acute ischaemia in the myocardium; in the second, arrhythmia is due to re-entry tachycardia in a scarred or hypertrophied myocardium. The mechanism in each group is different and further discussed in Chapter 4. It is difficult to assess the frequency of these two groups in relation to each other. Pathological series report a range of 20 to 80% for acute coronary thrombi in sudden ischaemic death (31,86). Studies of resuscitated cases of sudden ischaemic death also report evidence of acute myocardial ischaemia in 20 to 80% of patients (Table 2.2). The prognosis of patients who are resuscitated from sudden death due to acute ischemia is predicted to be better than those who have a chronic tendency to arrhythmias because of ventricular scarring.

Table 2.2 Clinical evidence of new acute myocardial ischaemia in resuscitated cases of sudden ischaemic death

	Q waves	Enzyme rise	Acute ischaemia	Ref
Goldstein et al.	44	34	78	(119)
Liberthson et al.	39	34	73	(120)
Baum et al.	19	38	57	(121)
Myerburg et al.	36		36	(122)
Cobb et al.	20.6	–	20.6	(123)

All figures are given as percentages

The discrepancies between clinical and pathological studies may be explained by differences in initial case-selection. It is possible to predict from the history which pathological process is more likely to be present. The absence of a previous history of ischaemic heart disease and, particularly, previous infarction with the presence of prodromal chest pain just before death, selects those with coronary thrombosis; sudden death in a patient with known previous infarction who has no chest pain in the last episode selects for a chronic ventricular arrhythmia. Thus, the proportion of each type is dependent on case-selection for entry to a study and, therefore, it is impossible to determine which type is more common. In a general survey of all sudden ischaemic deaths in a single community, 84.3% were thrombotic but, if only the subset of patients known to have had previous infarction were included, this figure was 22%. Exclusion of all patients with prodromal chest pain would ensure a series dominated by chronic arrhythmias (12). Angiography of the long-term survivors of out-of-hospital ischaemic heart disease and ventricular fibrillation shows Type II lesions in up to 30% (87,88).

Pathology of angioplasty

The morphological response to and clinical outcome of angioplasty is influenced by the nature of the lesion in terms of its tissue constituents and by whether it is a stable chronic lesion or an unstable plaque already undergoing spontaneous fissuring and thrombosis.

Pathological examination of successfully dilated chronic stenosis shows that splits extending to a variable depth into the intima at the lateral edges of the plaque are the usual mechamism by which the lumen is enlarged (89,90). Once the rigid intima is split, the media and adventitia allow further dilatation and the lumen is enlarged (91). The splits run deep into the plaque from the lumen and may reach the medial-intimal junction, although they do not usually extend far in this plane (Figure 2.28). Angiographically, these sites of successful angioplasty show an irregular outline and intraluminal haziness (90). A second mechanism involves eccentric plaques wherein the lumen is enlarged by stretching of the segment of normal vessel wall while the plaque itself remains unaltered. On angiography, these lesions appear to be smooth after angioplasty. In both instances, there is probably an element of outward shifting of the plaque through adjacent thinned media. If the intimal splits enter a large pool of extracellular lipid cholesterol, crystals may be extruded into the lumen or, more usually, forced outward through the thinned media into the adventitia.

There is a close analogy between the natural process of plaque fissuring and the intimal tears induced by angioplasty. Both act as a local stimulus for thrombosis because collagen is exposed to platelets. In angioplasty, however, the intimal injury and the thrombotic response are therapeutically controlled, and successful dilatation restores high blood flow, thus, limiting the development of thrombus. Some thrombus, however, inevitably forms over the collagen exposed in the intimal splits which, in turn, invokes the proliferation of smooth muscle cells which migrate into the area and lay down new collagen to restore a smooth outline to the vessel (92,93). Ultimately, there is regrowth of the endothelium into the arterial segment. It is not certain how long re-establishment of endothelial continuity takes but, in animal models, the intense thrombogenic potential of exposed collagen wanes after 24 hours, by which time the area is covered by a monolayer of platelets without an apparent tendency to invoke further adhesion and growth of the thrombus. It is likely that this reduction of thrombogenic potential of the exposed collagen also occurs in man.

Complications of angioplasty

The process of angioplasty is inevitably a stimulus for thrombosis and, not surprisingly, there is an incidence of early occlusion due to thrombosis. The risk is higher (94) with Type
II stenoses in unstable angina which already contain recently
formed thrombus as a potent stimulus to further thrombosis.

If the intimal tears extend too far, a dissection track may be
opened in the media into which blood passes, distally or proximally, thus forming an external haematoma which compresses
the lumen. The plane of the dissection track is the junction between the media and the adventitia, which has a natural tendency to cleave and allow blood to track. The greater risk of
dissection with Type II acute lesions (95) may reflect the ease
with which the angioplasty catheter can enter the intima, *via*
the rupture of the plaque cap, to reach the media.

There is also evidence that lipid-rich plaques without previous fissuring have an increased risk of dissection at angioplasty
(96). On dilatation of a lipid-rich plaque, the lipid is released
and the usual result is an outward spread into the adventitia,
producing a florid granulomatous giant cell inflammatory re-

Figure 2.28
Diagrammatic representation of the
sequelae of angioplasty.

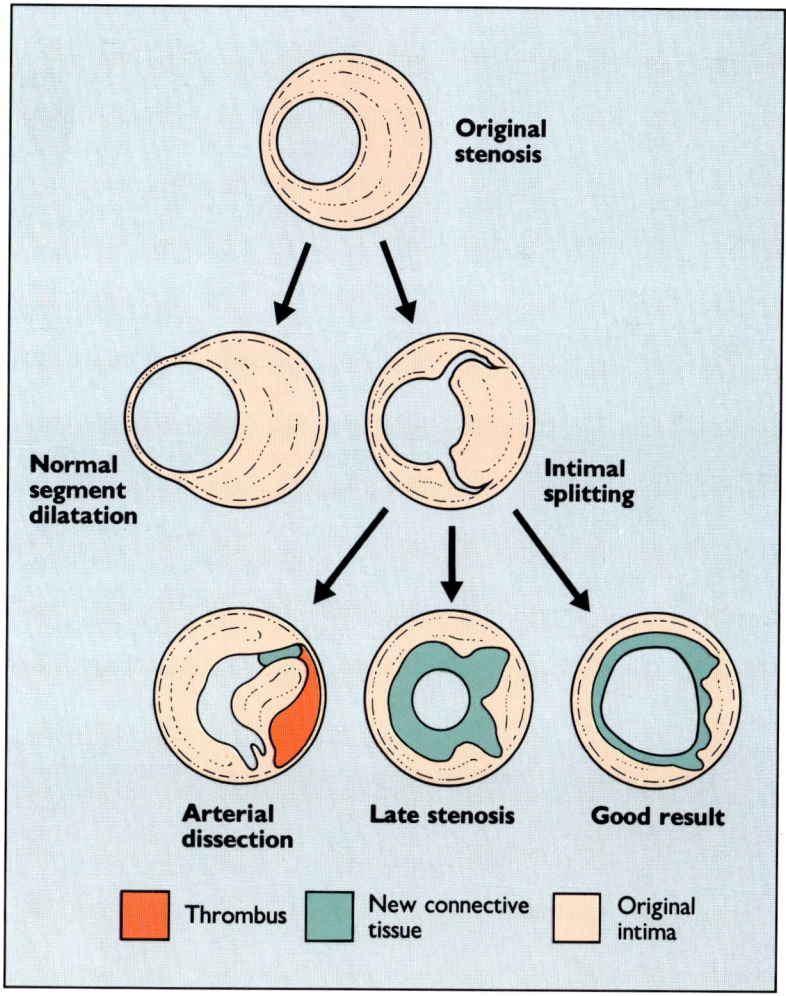

sponse. In some instances, however, appreciable amounts of cholesterol are extruded into the lumen and pass as emboli into the distal vascular bed. When large amounts of cholesterol are expressed, there is a granulomatous response in the myocardium with a close histological similarity to an area of myocardial sarcoid, but with the giant cell systems involving vessels. However, clinical evidence suggests that significant long-term obliteration of the distal vascular bed is rare (97).

The process of repair after angioplasty involves proliferation of smooth muscle cells and production of collagen (98) over a period of three to four months (18). The new collagen seals over the torn intimal flaps, forming a new concentric layer of fibrous tissue within the inner layer of the intima (Figure 2.28). Exuberant production of collagen in this layer leads to recurrence of stenosis at the angioplasty site in up to 30% of cases. Whatever the constitution of the original plaque, the new stenosis is predominantly young connective tissue which appears to be amenable to further dilatation, probably without further splitting of the intima. Redilatation is probably best carried out after the initial proliferation phase, when the new connective tissue has begun to mature (99). It is not certain what factors influence restenosis. Smooth muscle proliferation is at least partly dependent on growth factor released by platelets. It is very likely impossible, however, to prevent platelet activation after angioplasty, and growth factors produced by monocytes, endothelial cells and smooth muscle cells may be equally important. In experimental arterial injury, the early restoration of endothelial continuity over intimal tears has been shown to be an important factor in limiting smooth muscle proliferation at the site. The timing of the restoration of endothelial continuity following angioplasty in man is not known, but delay may be another factor in the pathogenesis of late stenosis.

Angioplasty of chronic occlusions

The majority of chronic total coronary artery occlusions are the result of organization of an occlusive thrombus related to an episode of plaque fissuring. The proximal portion of the occlusion is a complex mixture of dense collagen derived from the original plaque interspersed with loose connective tissue. More distally, the occlusion is mostly loose connective tissue and often contains several new vascular channels. If the proximal zone can be crossed by a guide wire, much of the distal occlusion can be easily dilated.

Pathology of thrombolysis

Arterial lesions

Consideration of the pathology of recent thrombotic occlusions shows:

> Three-quarters of acute thrombi result from plaque fissures;
>
> One-quarter result from more superficial injury without deep injury to the plaque.

An understanding of how thrombolysis restores blood flow can be derived from sequential angiography in living patients undergoing thrombolysis, and from reconstruction of the micro-anatomy of occluded coronary arteries, successfully or unsuccessfully reopened by thrombolysis, where the patient died within a few days from either cardiac rupture or cardiogenic shock.

Angiographic studies show that, after lysis restores a limited amount of antegrade flow, an intraluminal thrombus is revealed, which is then reduced in size more slowly until it finally leaves a complex irregular stenosis with some residual thrombus which is very resistant to further lysis (100,101). These data accord with thrombolysis reversing the thrombotic process in the same stages that led to occlusion. The thrombus formed in the final stage of occlusion is a lattice of fibrin filled with red cells and very susceptible to lysis; the second-stage mural thrombus comprises more densely packed fibrin and is likely to be more resistant to lysis. It is not certain whether lysis can remove the initial intraplaque component of thrombosis. Some morphological studies have shown that successful lysis may re-open the plaque, allowing further entry of red cells from the lumen, although this does not appear to be a significant factor in causing new acute occlusion due to plaque growth. It may be predicted from the known pathology of coronary thrombi that there will be considerable variation in the response to thrombolytic therapy (Figure 2.29).

Relatively few highly detailed pathological studies have as yet been reported (102). In some series (103), successful lysis was associated with the absence of plaque fissuring or with small plaque fissures but without a large intraplaque thrombus.

> Thrombolysis is more successful when plaque disruption is minimal.

Figure 2.29
Thrombolysis and the plaque structure
that underlies thrombi. Successful lysis
is likely in **A**, where the intraluminal
thrombus is the major component of
the occlusion. Lysis becomes more
difficult the larger the intraplaque
component becomes.

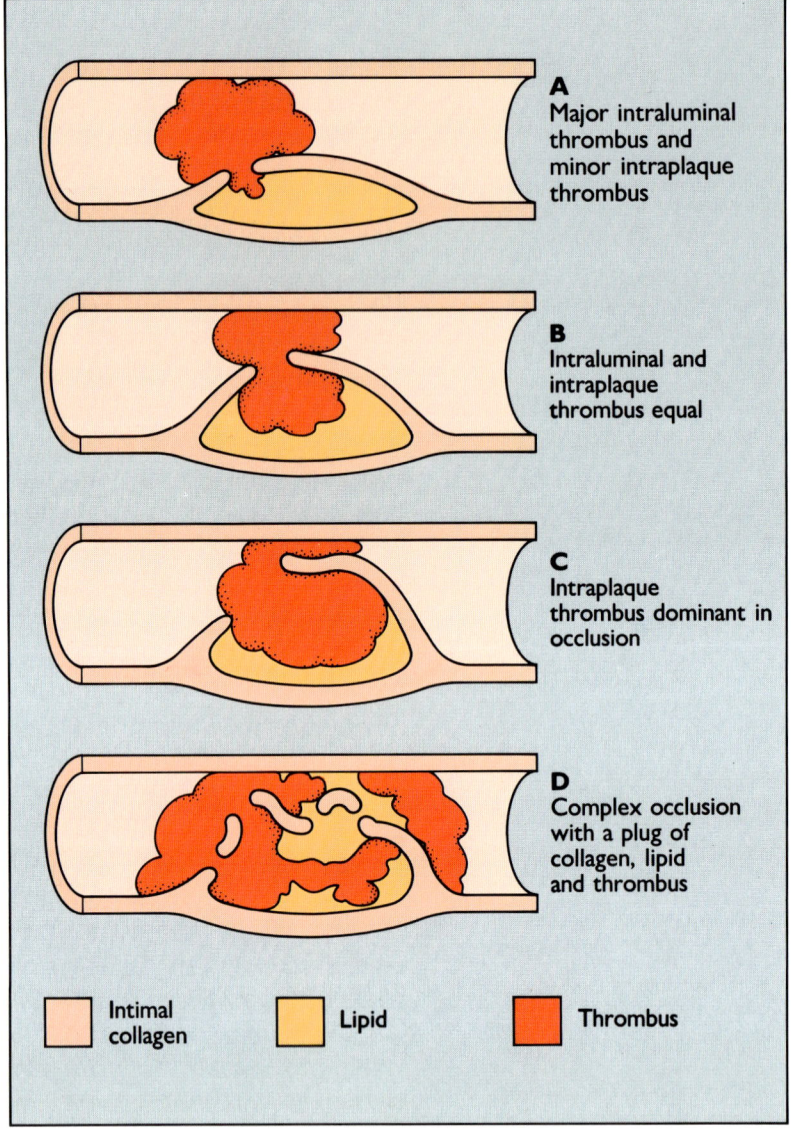

A
Major intraluminal
thrombus and
minor intraplaque
thrombus

B
Intraluminal and
intraplaque
thrombus equal

C
Intraplaque
thrombus dominant in
occlusion

D
Complex occlusion
with a plug of
collagen, lipid
and thrombus

Intimal
collagen   Lipid   Thrombus

Other series have shown that the majority of failed lysis is associated with complex plaque fissures (104). Some plaque fissures are major and extrusion of the plaque contents to form
a plug has been described in the failed lysis.

Unsuccessful lysis is associated with major plaque
disruption.

It may be that major plaque events require more specific
thrombotic agents, higher dosages, more local delivery of the
agent or associated angioplasty. There will always be a proportion of occlusions that do not reopen through lysis alone.

Angioplasty in association with fibrinolysis is the sole instance in which pathological studies suggest that extensive

intraplaque bleeding occurs, which may compromise the lumen more distally by compression from a subadventitial haematoma (105). Rethrombosis arises in 9 to 20% of successfully reopened vessels (106). Two factors, the presence of residual thrombus and high-grade obstruction, have been identified as indicating a high risk of reocclusion. Residual thrombus exposed to the lumen is perhaps the most potent known stimulus for further platelet activation. Residual high-grade stenosis is due both to the size of the original plaque and the extent to which it has been expanded by thrombus contained within it. Both causes of residual stenosis can be relieved by angioplasty, although the risk of dissection and haemorrhage is higher than when treating stable plaques.

Myocardial changes resulting from thrombolysis

Thrombolysis often re-establishes blood flow into an area of myocardium which has already undergone infarction. Such reperfusion alters the morphological appearances considerably; the most striking feature is intramyocardial haemorrhage (Figure 2.30). A vast majority of regional infarcts in patients who have not undergone thrombolysis are 'anaemic' in that they appear as yellow necrotic tissue at post-mortem examination; less than 5% show areas of haemorrhage. In contrast (105), the infarct zone in patients who have had successful thrombolysis is bright red (haemorrhagic infarction) in over 90% of cases. Histological examination shows the appearances to be due to extravasated red cells between the dead myocytes. The most straightforward explanation for the phenomenon is that damaged blood vessels within the infarct are reperfused, allowing extravasation of red cells. Identical appearances are seen following reperfusion of infarcted myocardium on inser-

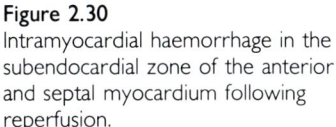

Figure 2.30
Intramyocardial haemorrhage in the subendocardial zone of the anterior and septal myocardium following reperfusion.

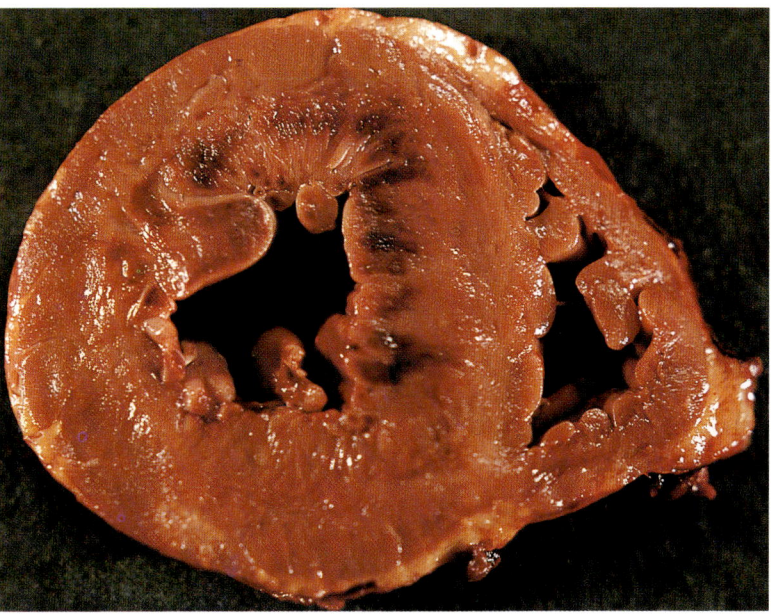

tion of saphenous vein grafts. The histological appearance of the dead myocytes is also altered to show contraction band necrosis instead of the 'coagulative' necrosis of non-reperfused regional infarction.

Changes in the appearance of an infarct is of no consequence unless it alters the clinical outcome. Individual cases have been reported in the literature where angiography has demonstrated intramyocardial pooling of blood following thrombolysis; it has been postulated that haemorrhage extends beyond the original infarct zone into normal myocardium and is a factor in depressing left ventricular function (105,107). Detailed pathological studies in man and in animal models of reperfusion of infarcted myocardium, however, do not support the view that haemorrhage occurs beyond the original infarct area (108).

It has also been proposed that invasion of the infarct tissue by fibroblasts is delayed in areas where haemorrhage has occurred (108). Evidence of this cannot be provided in man as it is not possible to ascertain the exact age of an infarct. The reports comparing two 'simultaneous' infarcts in one patient, only one of which was reperfused, are therefore not convincing. Furthermore, animal models have not supported delayed healing in haemorrhagic infarction (110).

The hypothesis that healing may be delayed after thrombolysis led to the suggestion of an increased risk of external rupture. The risk of late rupture following infarct expansion may be increased if haematoma formation within the myocardium was enhanced following an endocardial tear. Although the mechanism by which the risk of early rupture is increased is conjectural, it is far from certain that the risk of rupture is increased (102). There was a slight increase in the proportion of early deaths due to external rupture in some of the thrombolytic trials (111), but it is far from certain that this was absolute or relative, due to a reduction in infarct size and deaths from cardiogenic shock.

Coronary ostial stenosis

The majority of ostial stenoses occur in association with stenosis due to atherosclerosis at other sites in the coronary arteries. There is a small subgroup of patients, predominantly women without the classical risk factors for atherosclerosis, who have ostial stenosis as the sole angiographic lesion. The few pathological studies available, however, suggest that this subgroup has an unusual distribution of atherosclerosis rather than a dysplastic aortic root (112).

Infarction with normal coronary arteriograms

The reported frequency of regional infarction in which the sub-tending artery was angiographically normal ranges from 1 to 3% (113). There are several possible explanations for this (see Box).

Embolic occlusion: Emboli often lyse, leaving a normal artery, but it is clinically recognized that there was a potential source.

There was a minor acute plaque event with an associated thrombus which has lysed: The plaques which undergo fissuring are not necessarily large; when there is a small intraplaque thrombus and a large intraluminal thrombus, the lesion may resolve to angiographic normality. The excessive thrombotic response may be indicative of enhanced thrombogenesis or decreased lysis.

A previous coronary artery dissection has resolved.

Pure arterial spasm: It is now known that the use of cocaine may be an initiating factor (114), although many cases, particularly in younger women, were reported before the introduction of drug abuse and may not be due to this factor.

Coronary artery bridging: There is sound evidence in invidual cases of an association of myocardial bridging with infarction in the involved coronary artery; this may be recognized on arteriography (115).

There are no detailed pathological studies of more than individual cases from which estimates of the relative frequency of each cause of infarction in an angiographically normal artery can be made.

Coronary artery dissection

There is a steady flow of reported cases (116) demonstrating the angiographic pathological and clinical features of coronary dissection (see Box).

The plane of dissection in the coronary arteries is more superficial than in aortic dissection, occurring in the adventitial/medial junction rather than within the media itself. The adventitia contains an excessive number of inflammatory cells.

An intimal tear is sometimes absent and the lesion resembles a subadventitial haematoma compressing the lumen from outside. This form may rapidly revert to a normal angiogram.

There is a preponderance of female cases and an association with pregnancy.

Marfan's disease and 'cystic medial necrosis' are not usually present.

Angiography in a patient with a dissection may invoke dissection at another site. Even in cases not associated with pregnancy, there is some evidence of the risk being phasic.

A proportion of dissections associated with arteriograms carried out without technical difficulty may represent patients who are prone to spontaneous dissection.

Atherosclerosis in coronary grafts

Saphenous vein grafts universally develop a proliferation of smooth muscle cells within the intima a few days after insertion, providing that blood flow is established. This neointima is concentric and contains fine elastic fibrils embedded in a fibrous stroma. The intimal proliferation is normally self-limiting and does not encroach on the lumen. Smooth muscle proliferation may be a response to altered haemodynamic forces in the systemic circulation or may be initiated by platelet – endothelial reaction. Severe endothelial damage is inevitable, considering the methods used to harvest the veins, and all grafts show extensive platelet deposition over denuded endothelium in the first few days after insertion. Intimal proliferation may be sufficiently exuberant to cause focal stenosis at sites of anastomoses or ligature of side branches but, overall, is not a long-term cause of graft failure. The process is analogous to that found after angioplasty, and it is a moot point as to whether it should be regarded as atherosclerosis or a response to intimal injury.

Examination of patent venous grafts *post mortem* within a week of insertion shows most to have small thrombi within valve pockets and platelet deposition on the damaged endothelial surface. Any graft within which flow is not well established will completely thrombose. Atherosclerosis develops within venous grafts after several years (117) and is characterized by the accumulation of numerous lipid-filled foam cells within the superficial layer of the neointima. The deeper layer of the intima is not affected. Endothelial continuity is lost and thrombus becomes admixed with the foam cells to eventually occlude the lumen with a friable mixture of cholesterol and thrombus. The process is not focal but very uniform and diffuse, and plaque formation with localized stenoses is rare. The inner lining of affected grafts is very friable and any manipulation carries a high risk of embolism.

Internal mammary arterial grafts develop a minimal thickening of the intima which is easily offset by the steady increase in luminal size within the first few months after insertion. It does not appear that any form of atherosclerosis develops in internal mammary grafts within the time intervals followed so far, and their patency is superior to that of venous grafts of equivalent age.

Coronary artery aneurysms

The angiographic distinctions between coronary artery aneurysms, namely, localized bulges, local aneurysmal dilatation and generalized coronary artery ectasia, are not clearly defined. In the United Kingdom, the entire spectrum is usually described in relation to atherosclerosis. In atherosclerosis, the media behind a plaque usually vanishes: If the atheroma is evenly distributed, there is a uniform loss of media; if intimal smooth muscle proliferation is not pronounced, there is an area of arterial dilatation rather than stenosis. It is common for segments of stenosis to alternate with areas of ectasia in the coronary arteries; assessment of the stenosis is difficult because of the absence of an adjacent normal reference segment of artery.

The diffuse atheroma associated with ectasia is almost always associated with calcification in the deep layers of the intima. This calcification is, however, still intimal and there is no condition in the coronary arteries analogous to Monckeberg's sclerosis in the lower limb arteries.

Aneurysmal dilatation of an artery due to high blood flow occurs when there are anomalous origins from the pulmonary artery or when there is a shunt between the coronary artery and the coronary sinus, ventricle or atrium. In time, these dilated arteries develop diffuse atheroma and there is no structural difference from ectasia.

Medial destruction also results from acute arteritis; the most frequent cause is Kawasaki disease. In the acute phase, there is a significant mortality from thrombosis of the affected coronary artery; long-term survivors, however, develop both localized saccular and more diffuse aneurysms. In countries such as

Japan, where Kawasaki disease is endemic, older patients who present with coronary aneurysms are considered to have had a subclinical acute stage. The acute disease is seen sporadically in Europe and the United States, and it is possible that a few cases of coronary ectasia or aneurysm formation in these geographic areas are also the end-stage of an arteritis (118).

References

1. Singh RN. Progression of coronary atherosclerosis. Clues to pathogenesis from serial coronary angiography. *Br Heart J* 1984; 52: 451-61.

2. Haft JI, Haik BJ, Goldstein JE, Brodyn NE. Development of significant coronary artery lesions in areas of minimal disease. A common mechanism for coronary disease progression. *Chest* 1988; 94: 731-6.

3. Barger AC, Beeuwkes R, Lainey LL, Silverman KJ. Hypothesis: Vasa vasorum and neovascularisation of human coronary arteries. A possible role in the pathophysiology of atherosclerosis. *N Engl J Med* 1985; 310: 363-73.

4. Parums DV, Chadwick DR, Mitchinson MJ. Localisation of immunoglobulin G in chronic periaortitis. *Atherosclerosis* 1986; 61: 117-23.

5. Tracy RE, Kissling GE. Comparison of human population for histologic features of atherosclerosis. *Arch Pathol Lab Med* 1988; 112: 1056-65.

6. Tracy RE, Devaney K, Kissling GE. Characteristics of the plaque under a coronary thrombus. *Virchows Arch (Pathol Anat)* 1985; 405: 411-27.

7. Richardson P, Davies MJ, Born G. Plaque fissuring – the role of plaque configuration and circumferential stress distribution. *Lancet* 1989; ii: 941-4.

8. Mitchinson MJ, Ball RY. Macrophages and atherogenesis. *Lancet* 1987; ii: 146-9.

9. Faggiotto A, Ross R. Studies of hypercholesterolaemia in non-human primates. II. Fatty streak conversion to fibrous plaque. *Arteriosclerosis* 1984; 4: 341-56.

10. Davies MJ, Woolf N, Rowles PM, Pepper J. Morphology of the endothelium over atherosclerotic plaques in human coronary arteries. *Br Heart J* 1988; 60: 459-64.

11. Fuster V, Stein B, Badimon L, Chesebro JH. Antithrombotic therapy after myocardial reperfusion in acute myocardial infarction. *J Am Coll Cardiol* 1988; 12A: 78-84.

12. Davies MJ, Bland JM, Hangartner JWR, Angelini A, Thomas AC. Factors influencing the presence or absence of acute coronary artery thrombi in sudden ischaemic death. *Eur Heart J* 1989; 10: 203-8.

13. Uchida Y, Tomaru T, Kato A, Sonoki II, Tsuneaki S. Angioscopy of blood flow through stenotic arteries: Rheologic mechanism of thrombosis. *Am Heart J* 1987; 114: 1504-5.

14. Ross R. The pathogenesis of atherosclerosis – an update. *N Engl J Med* 1986; 314: 488-99.

15. Brown BG, Bolson EL, Dodge HT. Dynamic mechanisms in human coronary stenosis. *Circulation* 1984; 70: 917-22.

16. Epstein SE, Cannon RO, Talbot TL. Hemodynamic principles in the control of coronary blood flow. *Am J Cardiol* 1985; 56E: 4-10.

17. Serruys PW, Luijten HE, Beatt KJ, et al. Incidence of restenosis after successful coronary angioplasty: A time related phenomenon. *Circulation* 1988; 77: 361-71.

18. Roberts WC. The coronary arteries and left ventricle in clinically isolated angina pectoris – a necropsy analysis. *Am J Med* 1979; 67: 792-9.

19. Hangartner JRW, Charleston AJ, Davies MJ, Thomas AC. Morphological characteristics of clinically significant coronary artery stenosis in stable angina. *Br Heart J* 1986; 56: 501-8.

20. Freudenberg H, Lichtlen PR. Das normale Wandsegment bei Koronartstemon, eine post mortale studie. *Z Kardiol* 1981; 70: 863-9.

21. Saner HE, Gobel FL, Salomonowitz E, Erlien DA, Edwards JE. The disease-free wall in coronary atherosclerosis: Its relation to degree of obstruction. *J Am Coll Cardiol* 1985; 6: 1096-9.

22. Lichtlen PR, Rafflenbeul W, Freudenberg H. Patho-anatomy and function of coronary obstructions leading to unstableangina pectoris – anatomical and angiographic studies. In: Hugenholtz PG, Goldman BS, eds. *Unstable Angina*. Stuttgart: Schattauer, 1985: 81-94.

23. Von Arnim T. Eccentric coronary stenosis: A marker for spontaneous transient myocardial ischaemic attacks. *Br Heart J* 1990; (in press).

24. Mohiaddin RH, Firmin DN, Underwood SR, et al. Chemical shift magnetic resonance imaging of human atheroma. *Br Heart J* 1989; 62: 81-9.

25. Ambrose JA, Winters SL, Stern A, et al. Angiographic morphology and the pathogenesis of unstable angina. *J Am Coll Cardiol* 1985; 5: 609-16.

26. Bresnahan DR, Davies JL, Holmes DR, High HC. Angiographic occurrence and clinical correlates of intraluminal coronary artery thrombus: Role of unstable angina. *J Am Coll Cardiol* 1985; 6: 285-9.

27. Gotoh K, Minamino T, Katoh O, et al. The role of intracoronary thrombus in unstable angina: Angiographic assessment and thrombolytic therapy during ongoing anginal attacks. *Circulation* 1988; 77: 526-34.

28. Freeman MR, Williams AE, Chisholm RJ, Armstrong PW. Intracoronary thrombus and complex morphology in unstable angina. Relation to timing of angiography and in hospital cardiac events. *Circulation* 1989; 80: 17-23.

29. Forrester JS, Litvak F, Grundfest W, Hickey A. A perspective of coronary disease seen through the arteries of a living man. *Circulation* 1987; 75: 505-13.

30. Levin DC, Fallon JT. Significance of the angiographic morphology of localised coronary stenoses. Histopathological correlates. *Circulation* 1982; 66: 316-20.

31. Davies MJ, Thomas AC. Thrombosis and acute coronary artery lesions in sudden cardiac ischemic death. *N Engl J Med* 1984; 310: 1137-40.

32. Falk E. Unstable angina with fatal outcome: Dynamic coronary thrombosis leading to infarction and/or sudden death. *Circulation* 1985; 71: 699-708.

33. Fuster V, Chesebro JH. Mechanisms of unstable angina. *N Engl J Med* 1986; 315: 1023-4.

34. Bashour TT, Myler RK, Andreae GE, Stertzer SH, Clark DA, Ryan CJM. Current concepts in unstable myocardial ischemia. *Am Heart J* 1988; 115: 850-61.

35. Hackett D, Davies G, Chierchia S, Maseria A. Intermittent coronary occlusion in acute myocardial infarction: value of combined thrombolytic and vasodilator therapy. *N Engl J Med* 1987; 317: 1055-9.

36. Davies MJ, Thomas AC, Knapman PA, Hangartner JR. Intramyocardial platelet aggregation in patients with unstable angina suffering sudden ischaemic death. *Circulation* 1986; 73: 418-27.

37. Fitzgerald DJ, Roy L, Catella F, FitzGerald GA. Platelet activation in unstable coronary disease. *N Engl J Med* 1986; 315: 983-8.

38. Hamm CW, Lorenz RL, Bleifeld W, Kupper W, Wober W, Weber PC. Biochemical evidence of platelet activation in patients with persistent unstable angina. *J Am Coll Cardiol* 1987; 10: 998-1004.

39. Holmes DR, Hartzler GO, Smith HC, Fuster V. Coronary artery thrombosis in patients with unstable angina. *Br Heart J* 1981; 45: 411-6.

40. Nakagawa S, Hanada Y, Koiwaya Y, Tanaka K. Angiographic features

in the infarct related artery after intracoronary urokinase followed by prolonged anticoagulation. Role of ruptured atheromatous plaque and adherent thrombus in acute myocardial infarction in vivo. *Circulation* 1988; 78: 1335–44.

41. Vanhoutte PM, Shimokawa H. Endothelium-derived relaxing factor and coronary vasospasm. *Circulation* 1989; 80: 1-9.

42. Ludmer PL, Selwyn AP, Shook TL, et al. Paradoxical vasoconstriction induced by acetylcholine in atherosclerotic coronary arteries. *N Engl J Med* 1986; 315: 1046.

43. Palmer RMJ, Ferrige AG, Moncada S. Nitric oxide release accounts for the biological activity of EDRF. *Nature* 1987; 327: 524-7.

44. Maseri A. Role of coronary artery spasm in symptomatic and silent myocardial ischaemia. *J Am Coll Cardiol* 1987; 9: 249-62.

45. Brown BG. Observations linking the clinical spectrum of ischemic heart disease to the dynamic pathology of coronary atherosclerosis. *Arch Intern Med* 1981; 141: 716-22.

46. Nabel EG, Ganz P, Jordan JB, Alexander RW, Selwyn AP. Dilation of normal and constriction of atherosclerotic arteries caused by the cold pressor test. *Circulation* 1988; 77: 43-52.

47. Forstermann U, Mugge A, Alheid U, Haverich A, Frohlich JC. Selective attenuation of EDRF mediated vasodilatation in atherosclerotic human coronary arteries. *Circ Res* 1988; 62: 185-90.

48. Shimokawa H, Aarhus LL, Vanhoutte PM. Porcine coronary arteries with regenerated endothelium have a reduced endothelium dependent responsiveness to aggregating platelets and serotonin. *Circ Res* 1987; 61: 256-61.

49. Lam JYT, Chesebro JH, Steele PM, Badimon L, Fuster V. Is vasospasm related to platelet deposition? Relationship in a porcine preparation of arterial injury in vivo. *Circulation* 1987; 75: 243-8.

50. Forman MB, Oates JA, Robertson D, Robertson RM, Roberts LJ, Virmani R. Increased adventitial mast cells in a patient with coronary spasm. *N Engl J Med* 1985; 313: 1138-41.

51. DeWood MA, Spores J, Notske R. Prevalence of total coronary occlusion during the early hours of transmural myocardial infarction. *N Engl J Med* 1980; 303: 897-902.

52. Stadius ML, Maynard C, Fritz JK. Coronary anatomy and left ventricular function in the first twelve hours of acute myocardial infarction: The Western Washington randomized intracoronary streptokinase trial. *Circulation* 1985; 72: 292-301.

53. Bertrand ME, Lefebvre JM, Laisne CL, Rousseau MF, Carre AG, Lekieffre JP. Coronary angiography in acute transmural myocardial infarction. *Am Heart J* 1979; 97: 61-9.

54. Koren G, Weiss AT, Hasin Y, et al. Prevention of myocardial damage in acute mycardial ischaemia by early treatment with IV streptokinase. *N Engl J Med* 1985; 313: 384-9.

55. Brown BG, Gallery CA, Badger RS, et al. Incomplete lysis of thrombus in the moderate underlying atherosclerotic lesion during intracoronary infusion of streptokinase for acute myocardial infarction. Quantitative angiographic observations. *Circulation* 1986; 73: 653-61.

56. Little WC, Constantinescu M, Applegate RJ, et al. Can coronary arteriography predict the site of subsequent myocardial infarction in a patient with mild to moderate coronary artery disease? *Circulation* 1988; 78: 1157-66.

57. Ambrose JA, Tannenbaum MA, Alexopoulos D, et al. Angiographic progression of coronary artery disease and the development of myocardial infarction. *J Am Coll Cardiol* 1988; 12: 56-62.

58. Erhardt LR, Unge G, Boman G. Formation of coronary arterial thrombi in relation to onset of necrosis in acute myocardial infarction in man. *Am Heart J* 1976; 91: 592-8.

59. Henriksson P, Edhag O, Jansson B. A role for platelets in the process of infarct extension. *N Engl J Med* 1985; 313: 1660-1.

60. Davies MJ, Fulton WFW, Robertson WB. The relation of coronary thrombosis to ischemic myocardial necrosis. *J Pathol* 1979; 127: 99-110.

61. Maseri A, Chierchia S, Davies G. Pathophysiology of coronary occlusion in acute infarction. *Circulation* 1986; 73: 233-9.

62. Spodick DH. Q wave infarction versus ST infarction. Non-specificity of electrocardiographic criteria for differentiating transmural and non-transmural infarction. *Am J Cardiol* 1982; 51: 913-5.

63. Gibson RS. Clinical, functional and angiographic distinctions between Q wave and non-Q wave myocardial infarction: Evidence of spontaneous reperfusion and implications for intervention trials. *Circulation* 1987; 75: 128-38.

64. Hutler SM, Fresnvyid RW, Flynn T, Yeatman LA. Non-transmural myocardial infarction. A comparison of hospital and late clinical course of patients with that of matched patients with transmural anterior and inferior infarction. *Am J Cardiol* 1981; 48: 591-601.

65. Piek JJ, Becker AE. Collateral blood supply to the myocardium at risk in human myocardial infarction: A quantitative postmortem assessment. *J Am Coll Cardiol* 1988; 11: 1290-6.

66. Hirai T, Fujita M, Nakajima H, et al. Importance of collateral formation for prevention of left ventricular aneurysm formation in acute myocardial infarction. *Circulation* 1989; 79: 791-6.

67. Skehan JD, Carey C, Norrell MS, de Belder M, Balcon R, Mills PG. Patterns of coronary artery disease in post infarction ventricular septal rupture. *Br Heart J* 1989; 62: 268-72.

68. Weisman HF, Healy B. Myocardial infarct expansion, infarct extension and reinfarction – pathophysiologic concepts. *Prog Cardiovasc Dis* 1987; 30: 73-110.

69. Fuster V, Halperin JL. Left ventricular thrombi and cerebral embolism. *N Engl J Med* 1989; 320: 392-4.

70. Meltzer RV, Visser CA, Fuster V. Intracardiac thrombi and systemic embolisation. *Ann Intern Med* 1986; 104: 689-98.

71. Davies MJ, Woolf N, Robertson WB. Pathology of acute myocardial infarction wih particular reference to occlusive coronary thrombi. *Br Heart J* 1976; 38: 659-64.

72. Dellborg M, Held P, Swedberg K, Anders V. Rupture of the myocardium – occurrence and risk factor. *Br Heart J* 1985; 54: 11-6.

73. Becker AE, Vanmantgem JP. Cardiac tamponade – a study of 50 hearts. *Eur J Cardiol* 1975; 3: 349-58.

74. Schuster EH, Bulkley BH. Expansion of transmural myocardial infarction: A pathophysiologic factor in cardiac rupture. *Circulation* 1979; 60: 1532-8.

75. Vlodaver Z, Edwards JE. Rupture of ventricular septum or papillary muscle complicating myocardial infarction. *Circulation* 1977; 55: 815-22.

76. Tibutt DA. True left ventricular aneurysm. *Br Med J* 1984; 289: 450-1.

77. Davies MJ. Ischaemic ventricular aneurysms: True or false? *Br Heart J* 1988; 60: 95-7.

78. Lascault G, Reeves F, Drobinski G. Evidence of the inaccuracy of standard echocardiographic and angiographic criteria used for the recognition of true and false left ventricular aneurysms. *Br Heart J* 1988; 60: 125-8.

79. Visser CA, Kan G, Meltzer RS, et al. Incidence, timing and prognostic value of left ventricular aneurysm formation after myocardial infarction: A prospective, serial echocardiographic study of 158 patients. *Am J Cardiol* 1986; 57: 729-32.

80. Vlodaver Z, Coe JI, Edwards JE. True and false left ventricular aneurysms. *Circulation* 1975; 51: 567-72.

81. Reeder GS, Lengyel M, Tajik AJ, Seward JB, Smith HC, Danielson GK. Mural thrombus in left ventricular aneurysm. *Mayo Clin Proc* 1981; 56: 77-81.

82. Hochman JS, Platia EB, Bulkley BH. Endocardial abnormalities in left ventricular aneurysms. *Ann Intern Med* 1984; 100: 29-35.

83. Nashimura RA, Schaff HV, Shub C, Gersh BJ, Edwards WD, Takik AJ. Papillary muscle rupture complicating acute myocardial infarction – analysis of 17 patients. *Am J Cardiol* 1983; 51: 373-8.

84. Wei JY, Hutchins GM, Bulkley BH. Papillary muscle rupture in fatal acute myocardial infarction: A potentially treatable form of cardiogenic shock. *Ann Intern Med* 1979; 90: 149-53.

85. Thomas AC, Knapman PA, Krikler DM, Davies MJ. Community study of the causes of "natural" sudden death. *Br Med J* 1988; 297: 1453-6.

86. Warnes C, Roberts WC. Comparison at necropsy by age group of amount and distribution of narrowing by atherosclerotic plaque in 2995 five mm long segments of 240 major coronary arteries in 60 men aged 31-70 years with sudden coronary death. *Am Heart J* 1984; 108: 431-5.

87. Lo YSA, Cutler JE, Blake K, Wright AM, Kron J, Swerdlow CD. Angiographic coronary morphology in survivors of cardiac arrest. *Am Heart J* 1988; 115: 781-5.

88. Stevenson WG, Wiener I, Yeatman L, Wohlgelernter D, Weiss N. Complicated atherosclerotic lesions: A potential cause of ischemic ventricular arrhythmias in cardiac arrest survivors who do not have inducible ventricular tachycardia? *Am Heart J* 1988; 116: 1-6.

89. Block PC. Mechanisms of transluminal angioplasty. *Am J Cardiol* 1984; 53: 69-71.

90. Waller BF. Morphologic correlations of coronary angiographic patterns at the site of percutaneous transluminal coronary angioplasty. *Clin Cardiol* 1988; 11: 817-22.

91. Editorial. The pathology of coronary angioplasty. *Lancet* 1989; ii: 423-4.

92. Austin GE, Ratcliff NB, Hollman J, Tabei S, Phillips DF. Intimal proliferation of smooth muscle cells as an explanation for recurrent coronary artery stenosis after PTCA. *J Am Coll Cardiol* 1985; 6: 369-75.

93. Essed CE, Brand M, Becker AE. Transluminal angioplasty and early restenosis. Fibrocellular occlusion after wall laceration. *Br Heart J* 1983; 49: 393-6.

94. Perry RA, Seth A, Hunt A, Shiu MF. Coronary angioplasty in unstable angina and stable angina: A comparison of success and complications. *Br Heart J* 1988; 60: 367-73.

95. Hollman J, Gruentzig AR, Douglas JS, et al. Acute occlusion after percutaneous transluminal coronary angioplasty – a new approach. *Circulation* 1983; 68: 725-32.

96. Potkin BN, Roberts WC. Effects of PTCA on atherosclerotic plaques and relation of plaque composition and arterial size to outcome. *Am J Cardiol* 1988; 62: 41-50.

97. MacDonald RG, Feldman RL, Conti CR, Pepine CJ. Thromboembolic complications of coronary angioplasty. *Am J Cardiol* 1984; 54: 916-7.

98. Mcbride W, Lange RA, Hillis LD. Restenosis after successful coronary angioplasty. *N Engl J Med* 1988; 318: 1734-7.

99. Ueda M, Becker AE, Fujimoto T. Pathological changes induced by repeated PTCA. *Br Heart J* 1987; 58: 635-43.

100. Harrison DG, Ferguson DW, Collins SM. Rethrombosis after reperfusion with streptokinase: Importance of geometry of residual lesions. *Circulation* 1984; 69: 991-9.

101. Isner JM, Konstam MA, Fortin RV, Lefebvre M, Salem DN. Delayed thrombolysis of streptokinase-resistant occlusive thrombus: Documentation by pre- and postmortem coronary angiography. *Am J Cardiol* 1983; 52: 210-1.

102. Davies MJ. Successful and unsuccessful coronary thrombolysis. *Br Heart J* 1989; 61: 381-4.

103. Richardson SG, Allen DC, Morton P, Murtagh JG, Scott ME, O'Keeffe DB. Pathological changes following intravenous streptokinase treatment in eight patients with acute myocardial infarction. *Br Heart J* 1989; 61: 390-5.

104. Onodera T, Fujiwara H, Tanaka M. Cineangiographic and pathological features of the infarct-related vessel in successful and unsuccessful thrombolysis. *Br Heart J* 1989; 61: 385-9.

105. Waller BF, Rothbaum DA, Pinkerton CA, et al. Status of the myocardium and infarct-related coronary artery in 19 necropsy patients with acute recanalization using pharmacologic (streptokinase, r-tissue plasminogen activator), mechanical (percutaneous transluminal coronary angioplasty) or combined types of reperfusion therapy. *J Am Coll Cardiol* 1987; 9: 785-801.

106. Fuster V, Badimon L, Cohen M, Ambrose JA, Badimon JJ, Chesebro J. Insights into the pathogenesis of acute ischemic syndromes. *Circulation* 1988; 77: 1213-20.

107. Little WC, Rogers EW. Angiographic evidence of hemorrhagic myocardial infarction after intracoronary thrombolysis with streptokinase. *Am J Cardiol* 1983; 51: 906-8.

108. Kloner RA, Alker KJ. The effect of streptokinase on intramyocardial hemorrhage, infarct size, and the no-reflow phenomenon during coronary reperfusion. *Circulation* 1984; 70: 513-21.

109. Mathey DG, Schofer J, Kuck K-H, Beil U, Kloppel G. Transmural hemorrhagic myocardial infarction after intracoronary streptokinase. Clinical angiographic and necropsy findings. *Br Heart J* 1982; 48: 546-51.

110. Althaus U, Gwitner HP, Bauer H, Hamburger S, Roos B. Consequences of myocardial reperfusion following temporary coronary occlusion in pigs: Effects on morphologic, biochemical and hemodynamic findings. *Eur J Clin Invest* 1977; 7: 437-43.

111. Yusuf S, Collins R, Peto R. Intravenous and intracoronary fibrinolytic therapy in acute myocardial infarction. Overview of results on mortality, reinfarction and side-effects from 33 randomized controlled trials. *Eur Heart J* 1985; 6: 556-85.

112. Stewart JT, Ward DE, Davies MJ, Pepper JR. Isolated coronary ostial stenosis:

observations on the pathology. *Eur Heart J* 1987; 8: 917-20.

113. Fox KM. Myocardial infarction and the normal coronary arteriogram. *Br Med J* 1983; 287: 446-7.

114. Zimmerman FH, Gustafson GM, Kemp HG Jr. Recurrent myocardial infarction associated with cocaine abuse in a young man with normal coronary arteries: Evidence for coronary artery spasm culminating in thrombosis. *J Am Coll Cardiol* 1987; 9: 964-8.

115. Felman AM, Baughman KL. Myocardial infarction: association with a myocardial bridge. *Am Heart J* 1986; 111: 784-93.

116. Movsesian MA, Wray RB. Post partum myocardial infarction. *Br Heart J* 1989; 62: 154-7.

117. Bulkley BH, Hutchins GM. Accelerated atherosclerosis: A morphological study of 97 saphenous vein coronary artery bypass grafts. *Circulation* 1977; 55: 163-9.

118. Brecker SJD, Gray HH, Oldershaw PJ. Coronary artery aneurysm and myocardial infarction; adult sequelae of Kawasaki disease? *Br Heart J* 1987; 59: 509-12.

119. Goldstein S, Landis JR, Leighton R, et al. Characteristics of the resuscitated out-of-hospital cardiac arrest victim with coronary heart disease. *Circulation* 1981; 64: 977-84.

120. Liberthson RR, Nagel EL, Hirschman JC, Nussenfeld SR, Blackbourne BD, Davis JH. Pathophysiologic observations in prehospital ventricular fibrillation and sudden cardiac death. *Circulation* 1974; 49: 790-8.

121. Baum RS, Alvarez H, Cobb LA. Survival after resuscitation from out-of-hospital ventricular fibrillation. *Circulation* 1974; 50: 1231-5.

122. Myerburg RJ, Conde CA, Sung RJ, et al. Clinical electrophysiologic and hemodynamic profile of patients resuscitated from prehospital cardiac arrest. *Am J Med* 1980; 68: 568-76.